D1569309

WHAT EVERY MAN
SHOULD KNOW ABOUT
HIS
— PROSTATE —

WHAT EVERY MAN SHOULD KNOW ABOUT HIS
PROSTATE

Monroe E. Greenberger, M.D.
and
Mary-Ellen Siegel, M.S.W.

WALKER AND COMPANY, NEW YORK

First published in the United States of America in 1983 by
the Walker Publishing Company, Inc.

Published simultaneously in Canada by John Wiley & Sons
Canada, Limited, Rexdale, Ontario.

ISBN: 0-8027-0725-4

Library of Congress Catalog Card Number: 82-20068

Printed in the United States of America

10 9 8 7 6 5 4 3 2 1

Library of Congress Cataloging in Publication Data

Greenberger, Monroe E.
  What every man should know about his prostate.

  Bibliography: p.
  Includes index.
  1. Prostate gland—Diseases. I. Siegel, Mary-Ellen.
II. Title.
RC899.G73   1983   616.6'5   82-20068
ISBN 0-8027-0725-4

In memory of
Charles Chetwood, M.D., incomparable teacher of
urologists throughout the world, and for many years
my chief at French Hospital
and
Arthur J. Greenberger, M.D., brother, friend, teacher
and my associate for forty-four years.

M.E.G.

In Honor of
Milton I. Levine, M.D., who came into our lives over
fifty years ago and took care of me and my sister, and
later our children, with patience, warmth, devotion and
pediatric wisdom.
and
Robert E. Gross, M.D., who, in 1948, performed the
surgical procedure that became known as our family's
"miracle," and has remained a dear friend to us all.

My love and gratitude to you both.

M.E.S.

In memory of
Charles Chetwood, M.D., incomparable teacher of
urologists throughout the world, and for many years
my chief at French Hospital
and
Arthur J. Greenberger, M.D., brother, friend, teacher
and my associate for forty-four years.

M.E.G.

In Honor of
Milton I. Levine, M.D., who came into our lives over
fifty years ago and took care of me and my sister, and
later our children, with patience, warmth, devotion and
pediatric wisdom.
and
Robert E. Gross, M.D., who, in 1948, performed the
surgical procedure that became known as our family's
"miracle," and has remained a dear friend to us all.

My love and gratitude to you both.

M.E.S.

ACKNOWLEDGMENTS

We are grateful to the following people who gave of their time and expertise to help us bring this book to you.

Herbert Brendler, M.D., Professor of Urology, Director Emeritus, Department of Urology, Mount Sinai School of Medicine, New York; President, American Urological Association, Inc.; Editor, Journal of Urology.

Irving M. Bush, M.D., Chairman, Division of Urology, Chicago Medical School.

Michael Carrera, Ph.D., Professor of Community Health Education, Hunter College (CUNY), New York; Chairperson, Sex Information and Education Council of the United States (SIECUS).

William Fair, M.D., Chairman of the Division of Urology, Washington University School of Medicine, St. Louis, MO.

Deborah Green, M.S.W., Department of Social Work Services, Mount Sinai Hospital, New York.

Ezra M. Greenspan, M.D., Clinical Professor of Medicine (Oncology), Mount Sinai School of Medicine, New York; Medical Director, Chemotherapy Foundation, Inc.

Elliot Leiter, M.D., Director of Urology, Beth Israel Hospital; Professor, Mount Sinai School of Medicine, New York.

Karen Martin, M.A., Human Sexuality Center, Long Island Jewish Hospital-Hillside Medical Center, New York.

Arnold Melman, M.D., Associate Director of Urology, Beth Israel Hospital; Associate Professor of Urology, Mount Sinai School of Medicine, New York.

George Nagamatsu, M.D., former Chairman, Professor, Department of Urology, New York Medical College, Valhalla, NY.

Hans E. Schapira, M.D., Clinical Professor, Acting Chief of Services, Mount Sinai School of Medicine, New York.

Sidney M. Silverstone, M.D., Emeritus Clinical Professor, Department of Radiotherapy, Mount Sinai School of Medicine, New York.

Norman Simon, M.D., Clinical Professor, Department of Radiotherapy, Mount Sinai School of Medicine, New York.

Moses Swick, M.D., Emeritus Clinical Professor, Mount Sinai School of Medicine, New York.

We are also grateful to those colleagues who encouraged and supported us in this endeavor, and made many valuable suggestions. They are: Claire Bennett, M.S.W., Gail Button, R.N., William Gersh, M.D., George Klein, M.D., Gonzalo Lopez, M.D., Helen Rehr, D.S.W., Gary Rosenberg, PH.D., Judy Spielberg, R.N., Joseph Trunfio, M.D. Special thanks to Kay Workman who for over forty years has so patiently explained procedures and given reassurances to patients.

We are particularly grateful to Michael Gribetz, M.D., Assistant Clinical Professor, Department of Urology, Mount Sinai School of Medicine, New York, for his time and expertise above and beyond all expectations.

MEG
MES

CONTENTS

x

FOREWORD

Quality, compassionate health care is a collaborative effort which requires the coordinated activities of many people. The patient and family place trust in the physician to bring together all the health care professionals and resources needed to ameliorate pain, suffering and illness.

The high technology of modern health care is frequently mystifying and frightening to the patient. Constraints of time often prevent physicians from explaining the medical procedures and helping patients deal with their fears.

Books like *What Every Man Should Know About His Prostate* contribute substantially to the demystification of illness and health care. Although not a substitute for the interaction between the social workers, physicians, patients and other health care professionals, a book can serve as a more permanent and readily available reminder of the facts. More important, it can help the patient anticipate and cope with his treatment during this difficult period.

Although written primarily for the patient and his family, this book will be useful to the entire spectrum of health care practitioners. It not only provides a source of knowledge presented in straightforward language, but also helps the health care worker to anticipate patient concerns and to respond empathetically to them. Physicians themselves can gain from the book a better understanding of patient and family concerns.

The book reflects the efforts of a dedicated physician and a social worker, working together to explain the psycho-bio-social effects of male prostate health and illness. It is written with candor and sensitivity and assists patients and families in understanding what is happening in the physician's office, in the hospital and afterwards. It thus contributes to increasing the patient's knowledge and helping to make him an effective participant in his own care.

I believe that every reader will profit from the authors' wisdom and clarity. Their book is a splendid example of the collaborative process of health care at its best.

Gary Rosenberg, Ph.D.
Director, Department of Social Work Services;
The Mount Sinai Medical Center, New York

PREFACE

Sharing his experience and expertise as a urologist, Dr. Greenberger has written an enormously helpful book for all men. It is written so clearly that any reader can gain a broad understanding of prostatic problems and how they can be resolved by modern medicine.

Statistics tell us that by the time a man is sixty years old, he is more than likely to have experienced some symptoms of prostatic disorder. Many patients first report their symptoms to their family physician or internist. Frequently, suspicion of trouble will arise during digital rectal examination of the prostate at a regular periodic medical examination (which every male over forty should have every six to twelve months). The physician makes a preliminary diagnosis and then refers the patient to a urologist for more detailed examination and diagnosis, all of which Dr. Greenberger explains with great clarity.

If a diagnosis calls for surgery, the patient may develop great concern about his condition. This anxiety is best relieved by open discussion between the patient, his family, the family physician, and the urologist, as Dr. Greenberger advocates.

Patients in the older age group who require surgery often have medical complications such as heart disease, hypertension, diabetes or chronic pulmonary disease. Therefore, when the patient is referred to the urologist it is imperative that the family physician or internist continue to care for the patient's medical problems and acquaint the urologist with the overall medical status. If prostatic surgery is indicated, the family physician will advise the urologist if the patient is well enough to undergo surgery. He will also confer with the anesthesiologist to be sure that the surgical and post-surgical course goes smoothly.

I am pleased that the book discusses at some length the sexual concerns that patients with prostatic disorders often discuss with me, and, most important, that it offers reassuring solutions to many of these problems.

What Every Man Should Know About His Prostate is a splendid addition to the patient-physician relationship. It presents the latest information on the diagnosis and treatment of the several categories of prostatic disorders and says it in terms that a layperson can readily understand. It describes the importance of cooperation between patient, family physician and urologist and addresses the fears and concerns that most men and their families experience regarding the prostate.

The reader seems to feel that Dr. Greenberger is speaking directly to him. This book will prove to be extremely helpful to anyone, man or woman, who is concerned about the prostate.

Harold Brandaleone, M.D., F.A.C.P.
Associate Clinical Professor of Medicine
New York University College of Medicine

1

THE PROSTATE

After practicing urology for more than fifty years, it's hard to imagine a prostate problem I haven't treated. Of course, each man's prostate condition seems special to him, but the variations in this area are in fact remarkably few. An expert can treat most prostate ailments effectively and with a minimum of discomfort for the patient.

Preventing prostate disorders, however, is another matter. The incidence of such disorders increases every year. Curiously, this increase is a direct result of the medical successes that prolong life, because the longer a man lives, the more likely it is that he will experience prostate trouble. According to some estimates, half of all men need to consult a physician about prostate discomfort at some time in their lives. Those men who live to the age of eighty almost invariably suffer, or have suffered, from some type of prostate disorder.

Although the causes of prostate trouble vary greatly, the symptoms remain strikingly similar, regardless of the cause. These symptoms are all too familiar to many men:

- Frequent or urgent need to urinate
- Discomfort or pain during urination
- Inability to maintain the usual urinary system
- Pain in the pelvic or rectal area.

1

It is important to know that one or more of these symptoms may be a sign of other disorders as well. For this reason, I urge men to resist the temptation to diagnose their own ailment. Instead, they should speak first to their family doctors. The doctor can do the preliminary examination, and then, if necessary, a urologist can be brought into the picture.

THE NORMAL STATE

Knowledge about the prostate is sketchy among most nonprofessionals. They might know that it has something to do with a man's sex life, and that it can affect urination, and they may know it is a gland—but that's as much as they know. True, the prostate is involved in sexual activity (although rather indirectly), and it can interfere with urination when the gland is diseased or enlarged. But every man (and woman, too!) should be better informed about the prostate because he will then have the power to prevent minor problems from becoming major ones, the ability to know when something has gone wrong, and the background for working with the physician in making decisions that will influence his physical and emotional future.

The prostate, exclusively a male property, is located next to the inner wall of the rectum, around the urethra and directly below the bladder. It is usually described as consisting of five lobes, part glandular and part fibromuscular. Most of the prostate is between the urethra and the rectum and can easily be felt by the physician when he inserts his rubber-gloved finger into the rectum during a physical examination. I wish I could advise men to perform regular self-examinations, as gynecologists and family doctors tell women to perform on their breasts.

But it's just not possible, unless the man is a contortionist. I know; I have tried.

In its normal state, the prostate is about the size of a chestnut, but it is shaped somewhat like a pyramid. Just as men vary in height and weight, so their organs vary in size, but generally the normal prostate is about an inch and a half to two inches at its widest and weighs about 15 to 20 grams (less than three-fourths of an ounce). Some enlarged prostates I have removed weigh up to 275 grams.

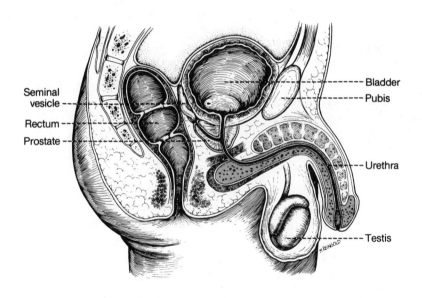

Seminal vesicle — Bladder
Rectum — Pubis
Prostate — Urethra
— — — Testis

THE GENITO-URINARY SYSTEM

CHANGING WITH AGE

The prostate is often likened to an apple with the core removed. The urethra, a muscular tube that carries urine from the bladder through the body and out through the penis, passes through the prostate, as the core would pass through an apple. Naturally, if the prostate becomes swollen, due to infection or to some disease, it will crowd the urethra and cause discomfort. Although the prostate is tiny in a newborn boy, it can be felt by the pediatrician upon examination, but apparently it doesn't begin to grow until puberty. At puberty the prostate is stimulated by male hormones and grows to its normal size. As a man nears fifty, the gland begins to grow again. No one is sure why there is more growth at that time of life. However, there is some evidence in dogs that it occurs because of an accumulation of dihydrotestostin, the breakdown product of the male hormone testosterone. Unfortunately, this change in size takes place at about the same time a man's sexual performance may be changing or declining. It's a time when he might have doubts about his ability to advance in his career; his children may be growing away from the family; his wife may be experiencing an uncomfortable menopause or developing new career interests outside the home. This period may be difficult for him in many ways, and symptoms of prostate enlargement (better known as benign prostatic hypertrophy, or BPH) only tend to exacerbate these concerns.

It is not at all uncommon nowadays for men to live into their seventies, eighties, and nineties without major medical problems. But because an estimated 60 percent of men over the age of sixty have some symptomatic prostatic enlargement, and up to 95 percent of eighty-year-old men have such a condition, doctors see more and more such patients. Cancer of the prostate is also on the rise because it usually attacks older men. Autopsies performed on elderly men whose cause of death is unrelated to cancer of the prostate add substance to the suspicion that cancer of the prostate is almost universal in men over eighty; but because of its slow progress and lack of overt symptoms, it is not often recognized. Infections, inflammations, irritations, and congestion are prostate problems that continue to affect males of all ages.

THE GENITO-URINARY SYSTEM

The prostate is actually a collection of thirty to fifty tubes or saclike glands connected to fifteen to twenty small ducts that are lined with a mucous membrane and surrounded by muscle and elastic fiber tissue. All of this is contained within a dense and fibrous "surgical" capsule. When someone says that he has had his prostate gland removed, it is likely that only some of the enlargement or growth has been removed, or perhaps that all of the glandular tissue has been removed from the capsule. Only in very special situations is the entire capsule removed.

This relatively tiny gland, which is capable of causing so much trouble, has few known purposes. Some doctors claim that the only function of the prostate is to produce a fluid for transporting sperm cells during ejaculation. It may have other functions, but they are not yet fully understood or defined. The prostate does produce enzymes, and perhaps hormones, too. Whether these enzymes and hormones perform any necessary function or contribute in any way to a man's general health has not been established.

The prostate does supply some of the seminal fluid, and its influence may be essential for sperm to function properly when it is ejaculated into the vagina. A male whose prostate gland has been removed is almost never able to impregnate a woman, even though sexual intercourse will be normal for him in every way. This may be due to the absence of prostatic fluid and to the result of the surgical procedure, which usually reverses the sperm's normal route. This procedure is described more fully in Chapter 8.

In all males, sperm travels a rather circuitous journey. It is produced in the testicles and takes approximately ten weeks to mature. At that time, sperm leaves the testicles and enters the epididymides (singular, epididymis), where it is stored for another three weeks. The epididymis is a tubular structure behind each testicle. After the sperm has matured, it travels through the vas deferens: a tube, or duct, attached to the epididymis. The two vasa deferentia (one from each testicle) loop behind the bladder, ending at points called ampullae. The sperm is stored in the ampullae until released through ejaculation. Next to the ampullae are the seminal vesicles. These saclike glands secrete a nutrient fluid (fructose, or milk sugar) needed to sustain the sperm. Connected to the seminal vesicles are the ejaculatory ducts that run through the prostate gland. The sperm and seminal vesicle fluid flow through these ducts, picking up nutritious fluid from the prostate, as well as fluid from the Cowper's glands (two pea-sized glands on either side of the urethra). This fluid then runs through the urethra and is expelled through the penis at time of ejaculation. About 95 percent of the fluid that is expelled is prostate secretion; about 4 percent is fluid from the seminal vesicles; and about 1 percent is composed of sperm and other secretions.

SOURCES OF PROSTATE TROUBLE

Much of what we know about the prostate has come to light since the end of the nineteenth century. The anatomy and physiology of the prostate gland were first understood at that time, and scientists realized that the prostate could become a site for cancer. However, four thousand years ago, the Egyptians treated the symptoms resulting from prostatic disease and abnormal growth. Even then they knew that a man who had to struggle to urinate, or was unable to urinate at all, was not only in great pain, but was also in danger of death. They inserted reeds, or copper or silver tubes, through the penis and urethra to widen the urinary passageway and allow urine to escape. This primitive catheter often turned out to be a lifesaver.

When urine is backed up in the bladder, crystallization often takes place and stones are formed. In ancient times, these stones were removed with these same crude instruments. The medicine men who performed the procedures later became known as lithologists (from the Greek *lithos*, meaning stone). Not until much later was the prostate itself recognized as the source of the problems. Its name is derived from both Greek and Latin, meaning "standing before."

Among the many problems a man can have with his prostate are enlargement, infection, and congestion. Enlargement (benign prostatic hypertrophy) usually occurs sometime after the age of fifty. Infections are often caused by bacteria that have traveled from other sites— such as teeth, sinuses, or tonsils—or by a past instance of venereal disease. Congestion can develop from various causes, among them a simple change in sexual habits. Although all these patients may share the same or similar symptoms, a treatment that is appropriate for one may be radically wrong for another.

Cancer of the prostate is, of course, a cause of more concern than all other prostate problems, but early detection followed by prompt treatment can be successful. Cancer of the prostate usually can be diagnosed before any symptoms are obvious; for that reason, I cannot stress enough how important it is for every man over age forty to have an annual (and later in years, semi-annual) rectal examination of the prostate by his family physician.

2
THE UROLOGICAL EXAMINATION

Fear of the unknown prevents too many men from consulting a urologist when they should. Often, a prostate problem can be handled so simply and so speedily that the patient is relieved of his discomfort before he leaves my office. Still, it is not uncommon for a patient to tell me that he has been suffering from symptoms of prostate trouble for months, even years, and has come to me because he just can't stand it anymore. Why stand it at all? A urologist can usually help.

All too often, a man waits until he has developed an acute retention before I get to see him. This means he is unable to urinate. It may happen in the middle of the night and often does. A man has had discomfort all evening, having to go to the bathroom constantly and just passing a few drops of urine. He doesn't call a doctor because he doesn't realize that he is going to be in real trouble soon. Because the passing of a few drops of urine offers relief, he thinks he's all right. But later—often in the middle of the night—he is unable even to release these few drops, and he is in real agony. If his own physician is unable to come over to his home and insert a catheter (a thin, smooth, flexible rubber or plastic tube inserted through the urethra and into the bladder to drain the urine), he is advised to go over to the emergency

9

room of his local hospital, where doctors there will treat him.

Sometimes I see a patient who hasn't urinated for twelve or fourteen hours, and I take out four quarts of urine. Usually this trouble occurs because of some sort of prostate obstruction, although there are other conditions that can cause it. It can also be caused by different drugs the man may have taken. Men in their sixties or seventies should not be taking antihistamines on a regular basis, because this can cause a contraction of the smooth muscle which surrounds the bladder neck and prostate, causing a urinary shutdown. This is usually not a problem in younger people, but anyone who experiences narrowing of the bladder neck and prostate may find antihistamines problematic. Too much alcohol, particularly beer, also can cause acute retention.

Most men who come to the urologist's office are not having an acute episode but have been sent by their family physician for a more complete diagnosis and possible treatment of a urological problem. Description of a typical urological examination as I perform it should reassure men about the relative painlessness and simplicity of the experience.

TAKING A COMPLETE HISTORY

The first thing I do, whether a patient has been sent by his family doctor or is self-referred, is to take a complete medical and social history. I ask him general questions about any illnesses or surgery he has had, and I ask him many specific quetions—such as whether there's been any swelling in his testicles, and whether he has ever had any injury to the testes or penis. I ask him how often he urinates and if there has been any change in his usual habits. Later, I ask him to urinate in my presence because, more often than not, a man's description of the urinary stream does not tell the urologist all he needs to know.

By observing the stream, I note whether it is a full, normal-size caliper stream, or if it is a thin stream that shows a narrowing which could be a stricture or a prostatic obstruction. If he has dribbling of urine or has to "push," this symptom suggests that the obstruction is somewhere in the urethra or the prostate. Sometimes I see what is called a split stream, where the stream seems to spray. That symptom is often due to a stricture of the external opening of the tip of the penis.

I ask a patient about his social habits—how much coffee and liquor he drinks. I also get a sexual history and ask him for details of his current sexual practices. Naturally, I ask him to tell me in his own words why he has come to see me, and I make a complete list of his complaints and symptoms.

As a rule, a man comes to see a urologist because he has pain in the area of the kidneys, back, or genitals, or because of some malfunction, discomfort, or pain he experiences during urination or sexual relations. Of course, in any particular case these symptoms may not be related to a urological condition at all, but the patient is in my office to find this out.

When a man is sent to me by his family doctor, I always ask for a detailed medical history from this doctor, too, including information on the patient's childhood diseases and any other infectious diseases he has had. I am interested, for instance, in whether he had rheumatic fever as a child, or nephritis (kidney disease). I am also particularly careful to look for any medical problems relating to the kidney if he had scarlet fever as a child, because kidney trouble was once a frequent side effect.

If he has ever suffered from enuresis (bed-wetting), that fact is also important.

I am particularly interested to learn if there is a history of diabetes in the patient's family. A predisposition to this disease often is inherited and may not surface until late in life. Diabetes can cause frequent urination, and it can cause sexual dysfunction. Sometimes I find that a patient who comes to me for urological treatment is really manifesting signs of diabetes. A complete urinalysis, which I do (and which the patient's family physician should also have done), will usually reveal evidence of diabetes.

WHAT URINALYSIS WILL SHOW

A urinalysis reveals much about a person's health. Among the abnormalities a urologist looks for in the urine sample are red blood cells, which suggest disease in the urinary tract, such as infectious prostatitis, benign prostatic hypertrophy, stones in the urinary tract, or tumors. These cells may also indicate tuberculosis. At one time, I saw many cases of tuberculosis of the prostate. It would begin in the lung or the bones and then travel to the prostate. Today, with the drugs that cure TB, I almost never see a case of prostatic tuberculosis, but it is still possible, so all urologists are careful to look for it. We also look for white blood cells or pus, which can indicate infection in the kidneys, ureters, bladder, or prostate. Urinalysis can also reveal sugar, which is a sign of diabetes; or albumin (protein substance) and kidney casts (fibrous material), which can indicate kidney problems. I also check the specific gravity of the urine to find out the number of solid particles it contains, an indication of the ability of the kidneys to absorb water and to secrete particles.

12

If the patient has any history of venereal or nonvenereal infections, I want to know, because these symptoms can cause strictures in the urethra and result in symptoms similar to those seen in prostate disorders. A full history of the man's surgical procedures is essential to me, and I will ask his medical doctor to share with me the findings from the patient's last complete medical examination. (A good medical checkup should include a routine electrocardiogram [ECG], a chest x-ray, blood chemistries, and urinalysis, in addition to a complete physical, including a rectal examination. I believe that every man should have a full checkup yearly, including a rectal exam, and after the age of fifty, a rectal exam twice yearly.) If a patient comes to me without having had such an examination and if he doesn't have a regular family doctor, I send him to a laboratory for an electrocardiogram and a chest x-ray.

I usually do a complete blood count (CBC) in my office. In the CBC, I look for departures from the normal standards, which may indicate general disease, and medical problems that may or may not be related to the urinary tract. Many doctors send their patients to a local commercial laboratory for these tests.

My staff does a complete urinalysis in the office, and, like most urologists, we do all our own x-rays of the urinary tract, too.

If the family doctor says, "Oh, aside from his urological problem, he's in good shape," and I am considering surgery (and even if I'm not), I request a more detailed report. Sometimes a patient may look well but has many physical problems. It reminds me of something my old friend, Mayor Jimmy Walker of New York, used to say: "You can walk by a building and the outside may be well painted and beautiful, but the plumbing inside can be in lousy shape." That holds true for people, especially

13

where urological problems are involved. A man may have a full head of hair, stand straight, and look like a healthy athlete, yet be running to the bathroom every hour due to prostate trouble. Most of the symptoms I have mentioned are very annoying and can interfere with certain life-styles. A truck driver, or a salesman who travels around town or has a long commute to work each day, will find the frequent need to urinate intolerable. But those men who have a bathroom near their office, and are seldom away from such a convenience for more than an hour or so, tend to ignore these symptoms. If a man needs to get up often at night, but he is someone who can fall right back to sleep, he may not be too troubled either.

If these symptoms have developed gradually over a period of time, a man may hardly be aware of them. Or he may think that it is normal at his age to have such problems. But it is not normal and, if ignored, can get worse and be that much harder to treat.

One symptom—blood in the urine—must *never* be ignored. If a patient says he voids some blood—even if he has no pain—I am concerned. The blood might be there only at the beginning of the stream; it might color the entire stream; or it might just be noticed at the completion of urination. In each case, it indicates something important. Although blood in the urine may be something other than a urological problem, it generally does show that something is wrong in the genitourinary tract or with the kidneys. Blood in the urine may be caused by anything from a simple inflammation to a stone or tumor. Painful hematuria (blood in the urine accompanied by pain during urination) suggests a stone in the urinary tract, or urinary tract infection, and of course must also have prompt medical attention.

X-RAY EXAMINATION

When a patient calls to make an appointment, my office staff schedules his checkup for the morning, and he is told not to eat or drink anything for twelve hours before his visit. The patient is also told to take an enema early that morning, if he has not had a bowel movement. The reason I ask this is that I may x-ray him. The x-ray requires injecting dye into a vein; this dye goes through the bloodstream and is excreted by the kidney. When the patient's fluid intake is withheld, his urine becomes more concentrated, so the dye can reveal more clearly the structure of the kidney, ureter, and bladder.

The x-rays of the kidneys, the ureter, and bladder show whether any stones have formed in this area, although uric acid stones are not readily visible. Because this x-ray is done after the patient has urinated, the picture will also show if there is a large residue of urine left in the bladder. If so, presumably there is an obstruction that is preventing the complete emptying of the bladder.

Next, a dye is injected intravenously (through the veins); it goes through the patient's body and outlines the urinary bladder, the ureters, and the kidneys. When the dye gets to the bladder, it shows any enlargement of the prostate. This intravenous pyelogram (IVP)—or intravenous urogram (IVU), as it is also known—consists of a series of pictures. The first x-ray film is taken within a minute or so after the dye is injected. Then, depending on what I see, I decide exactly how many more pictures to take and at what intervals. Generally I ask for four pictures taken ten, fifteen, twenty, and thirty minutes after the dye has been injected. If the prostate is greatly enlarged, the dye is delayed in passing through and will probably not show up in the early pictures. An obstruction of some other kind has a similar effect.

The use of contrast dye to outline body organs is used in numerous kinds of tests and was first introduced in the United States in 1929 by a young colleague of mine, Dr. Moses Swick. Dr. Swick had studied and performed research in Germany, and through his persistent efforts was able to develop the nontoxic intravenous drug that contributed so much toward urological diagnosis. The test, originally known as the Swick test, is now more commonly referred to as the IVP, or sometimes as intravenous urography.

Most people show no reaction to the dye. Others react mildly, but some people are strongly allergic to it. The dye has iodine in it, so I always ask the patient if he has an allergy to iodine. If a man tells me he is allergic to seafood (usually rich in iodine), I presume that he might suffer some reaction from the dye. When there is some question, I do a skin test for the allergy and then give a mild antihistamine.

Many urologists avoid giving an antihistamine to any patient they suspect has BPH because they want to avoid any chance of causing sudden urinary retention (inability to urinate). In all my years of practice, this problem has never occurred. Perhaps this is because I give such a mild dose of antihistamine, or it may be that I have just been fortunate. Some urologists simply avoid doing an IVP on such patients and use alternative methods for diagnosis.

Naturally, if a patient reports to me an experience he has had in another doctor's office or hospital where he had some test with contrast dye in which he had a severe reaction (chills, fever, and hives), I avoid the IVP. However, with the refinement of the intravenous fluid used today, there are few complications.

16

In those instances where I cannot do an IVP, where the IVP does not show the kidneys clearly enough, or where there is indication of abnormalities that need further investigation, I also do a retrograde pyelogram sonogram, or renal scan. Sonograms and most scans are noninvasive tests; that is, they do not require any material or instrument to be injected or inserted into the body. The retrograde pyelogram is the test that was used before the advent of the intravenous pyelogram. To do this test, I cystoscope the patient.

The cystoscope is a slim, hollow metal tube that is inserted into the penis and passes through the urethra into the bladder. At the end of this instrument, there is a light to illuminate the bladder interior. By means of a number of lenses, the urologist can see not only the inside of the bladder, but he can also get a close look at the entire lower urinary tract. There are various sizes and designs of cystoscopes to provide a choice for the one best suited to each individual patient.

Through the cystoscope, I introduce catheters into the right and left ureters and then inject a dye that outlines the interior of the kidneys. My experience has been that those people who are allergic to dye when injected intravenously are not allergic when the dye is introduced into the kidneys by way of the ureters. However, some urologists and radiologists feel this is risky, because under some circumstances an allergic reaction could be set into motion. However, the retrograde pyelogram is not a routine test. It is usually not painful—although it is more uncomfortable than the IVP—and is done in the office. The only anesthetic needed is a local one, such as Xylocaine, which is injected before the cystoscope is introduced.

The first visit to the office includes a thorough physical examination, which usually begins with the patient lying

17

flat on his back. This way I can palpate the lower abdomen to see if the bladder is full. I examine the kidneys thoroughly, then the abdominal wall. Then the patient sits up, and I check the skin of the back over each kidney, just under the rib cage, looking for areas of tenderness and for any enlargement.

A man's external genitals are examined most easily when he is standing. I examine the penis and the testes for any abnormalities or any signs of infection. I look for any possible cysts, growths, or tumors in the testicles and penis. I carefully check for a varicocele, an enlargement of veins which can cause a benign boggy tumor of the scrotum, and which recently has been implicated as a cause of infertility.

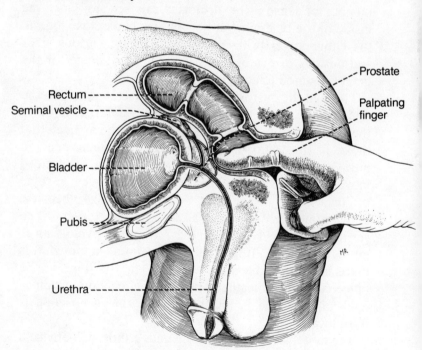

THE DIGITAL RECTAL EXAMINATION

DIGITAL RECTAL EXAMINATION

To check for any rectal abnormalities, for any ne
cal problems in the anal sphincter or the bladder
check the prostate itself, I ask the patient to ben
waist and lean over the examination table or chai
insert a well-lubricated index finger into his rectu
digital examination, as it is called, is the one pa
examination some men will object to, but it i
painful nor uncomfortable. Once a man has had
examination, he usually does not resist the next

The normal prostate feels smooth, elastic, a
the size of a chestnut. When affected by benign
hypertrophy (enlargement of the gland), the
feels similar but larger. Sometimes BPH canno
nosed by examination because the growth is int
of the bladder, but this will show up in the x-ra

The urologist, with his "trained" index fi
detect acute inflammation and any other disord
important, he can detect early signs of cancer
for a small hard nodule or areas of undue
(Chronic infections or stones can mimic th
malignancy, but infections can be determined
bacteria in the urine, and an x-ray will identify
I suspect cancer, I ask the patient to enter t
for a biopsy: a minor surgical procedure in w
of the hard nodule or other tissue is removed
snipping or by aspiration, and is then su
laboratory tests. No matter how convinced I
hard nodule is or is not cancer, I cannot be (
percent certain without laboratory proof.

Sometimes I have a patient who is hesitant
into the hospital, even though I suspect canc
"Well, I can live with this another month or
him, "I can only tell you that if you were my
pick up the phone now and get a bed fo

19

hospital. I can't do this because you are not my brother, but if you were, that's what I would do." That usually makes him recognize the importance, and he agrees.

If the patient is still hesitant, I say, "Well, if you have some business things that you want to take care of, do that, but I want you in the hospital within a week. Beyond a week, you take responsibility, not me." That usually does it.

Sometimes the news is good. It's not cancer or, if it is, it's at the very early stage and will probably respond well to treatment. (Chapter 7 will discuss the details of cancer of the prostate and the treatment available for it.)

CYSTOSCOPY

After the x-rays have been taken and I have performed a physical examination, if I feel it is necessary, I will cystoscope the patient. Many patients are frightened when I tell them I want to use the cystoscope on them because they have heard that it is a painful procedure. This is seldom so. I always inject some local anesthetic such as Xylocaine into the penis about fifteen minutes before I do the cystoscopy, and there is almost no pain at all. I always assure the patient that the local anesthetic I use will prevent pain, and that I will stop the procedure if he should feel the slightest discomfort. I believe all urologists and clinics use this local anesthetic—or should. If a patient is about to be cystoscoped without the anesthetic, he has good reason to protest.

Occasionally I get a patient who is so afraid of the cystoscope, even when I tell him it won't hurt, that I decide to do it in the hospital under general anesthesia. Cystoscopy is seldom necessary in a simple case of prostate enlargement, especially if the rectal examina-

tion plus x-rays confirm this diagnosis. If the prostate is extremely large, or if there's any blood in the urine, we want to determine by cystoscope if there is a tumor or any other abnormality in the bladder.

The initial visit to my office usually takes less than an hour from the time the patient arrives until he is fully dressed again and on his way. Generally, at this time, I am able to give him some idea as to what his trouble is. Also, depending on the diagnosis, we have probably decided on a beginning course of treatment.

If the patient gets a clean bill of urological health from me, his family doctor will probably run additional medical tests and refer him to the appropriate specialist to rule out any other disorders. Regardless of my findings, I always pick up the phone in the presence of the patient and speak to the referring doctor. I report to him about the tests and examinations I have done, and about what I have found. Later he will get all this in writing, but I think the immediate communication is helpful to both the patient and his family doctor. If nothing else, it reassures the patient that I have been truthful with him and that there are no secrets between the doctors about *his* body. My patients seem to appreciate this method, and I find, perhaps as a result, that they are usually very cooperative patients.

3

PROSTATITIS:
ACUTE AND CHRONIC

Inflammation of the prostate (technically, prostatitis) is so common that every man, from teenager to golden-ager, should be prepared for the possibility that it can occur in him at any time. Although prostatitis may at first seem serious to the patient, this condition usually responds well, if slowly, to treatment.

Infection, irritation, congestion, or a combination of these problems can cause prostatitis. The respective treatments vary, depending on the cause, the symptoms, and the personal habits of the patient. To begin, I will discuss infectious prostatitis, both acute and chronic.

Few problems will send a man to his doctor faster than acute prostatitis. Small wonder. In addition to numerous typical difficulties concerning urination (urgency, hesitancy, burning, pain, pus or blood in the urine), he may also experience low-back pain, nausea, vomiting, and fever. If his family doctor suspects acute prostatitis, he will probably send the patient to a urologist for confirmation of this diagnosis.

BACTERIAL INFECTION

Acute prostatitis is caused by bacteria that have found their way into the prostate. Unfriendly bacteria can

22

reach the prostate area via the bloodstream, the lymph system, the penis, and the urethra. So it's not surprising that an infection which seemed inconsequential where it began can turn up elsewhere in the body and cause very serious problems. The most common prostatic infection comes from colon bacilli. These bacteria reach the prostate either directly from the rectum or through the bloodstream. Fortunately, since the advent of antibiotics, this problem is less common than it once was. Even if an infection does take hold, it can usually be cured before it becomes too serious. Tonsilitis, an abscessed tooth, or a sinus infection are frequent causes of prostate infection. So are such infections as trichomonas vaginalis or candida albicans (yeast infection), which can be transmitted from a woman during sexual activity. Gonorrhea can also cause acute prostatitis. But some of the less dramatic sources of prostate infections include contaminated water systems, unsanitary swimming pools, and beaches.

Bacteria that find their way into the prostate gland discover a very hospitable host. The prostate resides in a capsule that is not easily penetrated and is fairly well protected against any infectious organisms in the system. But when such organisms *do* find their way in, they are often there to stay. Because the prostate does not drain itself well, the infection can easily take hold, and antibiotics do not always completely eliminate the organism from the capsule.

When the infection is acute (and usually the first time the symptoms are noticed, it is acute), it can often be cleared up with antibiotics, but a doctor should never say with certainty that he has cured it. These infections have a tendency to recur over and over again—chronic conditions, uncomfortable and bothersome.

Is there some way to prevent acute prostatitis? Sometimes, yes. Good health practices are important in pre-

23

venting any infection. When you hear, "Don't drink the water" about some foreign countries, take heed. Aside from the miserable stomach upsets that can result, contaminated water can introduce dangerous bacteria to any part of your body, including the prostate.

Certain substances in one's diet can cause a type of chronic prostatitis. Too much coffee is one of these foods, as are gin and highly flavored scotch whiskey and red wine. The flavorings in these drinks have a significant amount of aromatic oils that can irritate the prostate. Although these beverages are not likely to cause the initial attack of prostatitis, or even contribute to it, the weakened prostate is very susceptible to the effects of any highly spiced food or drink.

SEXUALLY TRANSMITTED INFECTIONS

If your sexual partner has either of the mild but annoying ailments, trichomonas vaginalis or candida albicans, she can transmit these to you. If they go untreated in the male, they can cause infections of the prostate. It is important to note that although these conditions of the female are sexually transmitted, they are not, in the usual sense, venereal disease. They can begin spontaneously in a woman and have no relation to her sexual practices or partners. Even a woman who has had no sexual experiences can and often does develop these conditions.

Women who develop such problems should be sure their partner knows about them because (particularly with trichomonas vaginalis, which may go unnoticed in the male) he, too, should be treated. These ailments tend to be passed back and forth between partners. Of course, if the infections travel from the penis through the urethra into the prostate, they can become much more than a nuisance. Any change that a man notices on his penis—skin eruptions, for example—should be brought to the attention of his physician at once. It might be something that can cause prostatitis if it is not checked at its inception. Some of these conditions can be treated locally with an antibiotic cream or ointment; others require oral medication.

At one time gonorrhea was the most common cause of all major infections of the male urogenital tract. Since the advent of penicillin, gonorrhea can usually be cured quickly, before it has a chance to travel to the prostate. However, I still see occasional abscesses in the prostate caused by gonorrhea, particularly among men who acquired some drug-resistant strain, and also among other men who have simply ignored prompt treatment. These patients exhibit the same general symptoms of acute prostatitis described earlier in this chapter. However, in performing a rectal examination on these men, I often detect a beginning abscess and severe inflammation in the prostate.

In the 1920s and 1930s, before modern drugs and antibiotics, the prostate abscess sometimes had to be incised. These abscesses were opened through the urethra by introducing an instrument through the penis right into the prostatic area. Although the infection didn't spread to other parts of the body and didn't kill the patient, it was capable of making him very ill. (Today if that occurs—and it rarely does—a doctor can surgically and painlessly incise it, entering through the rectum. It's a relatively minor procedure.) Most of these abscesses resulted from a gonorrheal infection. Although doctors couldn't cure gonorrhea with penicillin the way modern doctors do, they were able to treat infections by irrigating the urethra. They also used diathermy to treat infections of the urethra and prostate.

Diathermy is an electrical treatment rarely used today. The doctor would place one electrode in the rectum of a patient, touching the prostate gland. Another electrode was placed on the abdomen. Then the doctor would turn on the diathermy current. The main part of the heat generated would be concentrated between the two electrodes, thus focusing directly on the prostate gland. Since the advent of antibiotics, diathermy is no longer used in urology.

Sitz baths were frequently recommended in those days, and I still recommend them. A sitz bath is really just an ordinary hot tub bath, but the heat from the water as the patient sits in it has a therapeutic effect because it increases circulation to the affected area. Sitz baths have long been a good first-aid treatment for many urinary retention problems. I often suggest one when a patient calls me to say that he is having trouble urinating, unless he is in severe pain or in acute retention (pain from inability to urinate at all). Then I see him in my office as soon as possible. Sitz baths are also used, along with other treatment, for acute and chronic prostatitis, as well as for an enlarged prostate.

A favorite story of mine involves my coauthor, who at the age of nine was already practicing to be a social worker. One evening my wife and I had just returned from dinner, and we overheard the following phone conversation. My daughter was saying, "Oh, Mrs. Jones, I know your husband is in pain and I'm sorry, but my dad's out for dinner. Now if you will just run a nice hot bath for your husband and tell him to sit in it, he will feel much better, and by that time my dad will be home. He would only tell you the same thing and then remind you to bring your husband into the office first thing in the morning. But if you don't trust *me,* call back later."

26

DIAGNOSING AND TREATING ACUTE PROSTATITIS

When a patient comes to me suffering from what appears to be an acute prostatitis, I am very careful not to press on the prostate too vigorously while examining him, because too much pressure might spread the infection to the testicles, epididymus, or bloodstream. I merely palpate the prostate gently, in order to release some of the prostatic fluid for microscopic examination. This fluid is then expelled through the urethra and penis.

Various tests help the urologist to determine whether the patient's prostatitis is the acute or chronic, the congestive or irritative type, so the urologist must pay careful attention to the medical and sexual history of the patient. Past bouts with the same problem suggest to me that the patient once had acute prostatitis and is probably suffering a recurrence now. He is most likely someone who has had, and will continue to have, chronic prostatitis. Congestive and irritative prostatitis is usually due to certain sexual practices or to a change in habits. Infection is rarely involved in this kind of prostatitis, although it can coexist with all kinds of prostate problems. For this reason, both congestive and irritative prostatitis are sometimes difficult to diagnose accurately and treat effectively.

CHRONIC PROSTATITIS

Chronic prostatitis often follows a case of well-treated but not completely cured acute prostatitis, or it can simply exist without ever having become acute. It ranges from a mild state, almost symptom-free, to a state of extreme discomfort. Fever seldom accompanies chronic prostatitis. A man with chronic prostatitis feels an un-

27

comfortable fullness in the rectum, rather than pain, but it is certainly an unpleasant condition that must be remedied.

This ailment is frustrating for both patient and urologist because just when the patient begins feeling better, the symptoms start up again. Even the most loyal patient begins to wonder if he should see another urologist, and many patients do. However, any well-trained, ethical urologist they consult will explain that chronic prostatitis is often never really "cured," and that the best any doctor can often hope to do is to keep the patient comfortable and relatively symptom-free.

A man who has chronic prostatitis tends to worry that he is more likely to develop benign prostatic hypertrophy or cancer of the prostate than other men. On the contrary, he may have a better chance of avoiding serious trouble from these diseases since he sees a urologist regularly. In office examinations, the specialist is quick to recognize the earliest stage of BPH or cancer *if* it occurs.

Why doesn't a urologist end a case of chronic prostatitis by removing the prostate?

SURGERY SELDOM THE ANSWER

I often compare chronic prostatitis with tonsilitis. Some people get frequent mild attacks of tonsilitis, with an occasional acute attack. A doctor may say that they have chronic tonsilitis, but unless it is acute, doctors rarely advocate removing the tonsils. And, of course, they never remove them during an acute attack. They wait for the tonsilitis to subside.

In the same way, prostatitis seldom has to be treated surgically. Occasionally, if a case of chronic prostatitis

28

becomes intolerable to the patient, or if it causes urinary retention or kidney problems, surgery may be performed—but not during an infectious stage.

We may also continue with the analogy between tonsilitis and prostatitis by saying that some people seem to have a tendency to the problem. It is difficult to explain why, except to consider the problem their Achilles' heel. Doctors always hope that the latest antibiotic will be the one to offer a lasting cure for this persistent problem. They discover that the bacteria infecting the prostate soon becomes immune to the effects of the drug or that the drug is poorly concentrated in the prostate. One new drug, trimethroprim-sulfamethoxasole, better known as TMP-SMZ, is encouraging because it seems to offer long-lasting relief by achieving a high concentration in the prostatic tissue.

There is as yet no completely satisfactory drug treatment for prostatitis, and no urologist can promise a cure, but there is an effective treatment for chronic prostatitis. Most urologists will agree with me that symptoms can be greatly relieved by a doctor's massaging of the prostate at regular intervals. The physician simply inserts a gloved finger into the rectum and strokes the prostate very gently. Then later, as any remaining infection subsides, he strokes more vigorously. Massaging the prostate relieves the symptoms by draining accumulated prostatic fluid from the glands and ducts.

TREATMENT OF CHRONIC CONDITIONS

Naturally, the course of treatment varies among patients who suffer from chronic prostatitis but, generally, a prostate massage once or twice a week lessens the symptoms so that the patient may visit his doctor less frequently. Eventually, he can do without treatment for several months at a time. During this period, the man will be comfortable and so free of symptoms that he tends to forget that he has chronic prostatitis. He will go to work, sleep well, and remain as sexually active as he wishes without any problems. But his chronic prostatitis is often *not* cured; it is merely under control. I encourage such a patient to come in and see me at regular intervals, even if there are no symptoms, so that we can avoid a bad flare-up. Sometimes a man will call the office before his next appointment, complaining not of pain but of a sense of heaviness in his rectum and some feelings of pressure. I tell him to come in for an examination, and if there are no other problems, I give him a prostatic massage and he feels better.

Patients with chronic prostatitis become sensitive to recognizing symptoms of a flare-up in its earliest stages, and most of them call me before they are really miserable. I encourage this habit because I always feel that a patient who is alert to his own body is the best kind of patient I can have. I don't believe that people should try to treat themselves (even doctors mustn't do this!), but I believe that an educated patient is one who notices differences in the way his body is behaving and who knows when "something" is wrong, even if he can't be sure what that "something" is.

Once a patient came to see me, although his family doctor had assured him everything was all right. He said that he suffered neither pain in the pelvic area nor any urinary tract symptoms. However, he said he felt a general "heaviness" in his pelvic and genital area. Something told him this wasn't normal. Initially, my examination didn't reveal any problems, but the IVP showed a large prostatic stone. It hadn't yet given him any serious trouble, but it might have done so very soon. He was wise to be "stubborn" about seeking help for what he knew was not "right" with his body.

My coauthor, who is a social worker, says that she encourages people to trust their instincts about emotional situations because these so-called instincts are really a response to some unconscious learned experience. If you instinctively feel that something is wrong with your body, trust those instincts and call your doctor. If he isn't willing to listen carefully to you, and to ask questions and give you a careful examination, you ought to change doctors. No one knows better than you if your body isn't working right. However, don't rely *only* on your feelings about yourself. Get regular checkups too. Many things can go wrong with your body long before there are symptoms.

Perhaps more than anything else, a patient with chronic prostatitis must learn not to expect quick results. He may notice some improvement after only a visit or two, but it often takes much longer. Treatment may go on for months, even years.

While I am treating a patient, I also watch him for any other prostatic problems, and for any other ailments that may be due directly or indirectly to his prostatitis. Sometimes a man who has frequent infections of the prostate has a tendency to develop stones in the gland, which then perpetuates infection, so that surgery may be required to remove these stones. The surgery will probably be closed surgery, a fairly simple technique called transurethral resection, or TUR. This procedure is described in detail in Chapter 6.

Recently there has been some discussion among urologists and nutritionists about the effects of zinc in the body, and particularly about its effect on prostatic problems, especially enlargement of the prostate gland (benign prostatic hypertrophy). It is possible that zinc may be helpful in treating chronic prostatitis as well. Chapter 8 will discuss this issue in some detail.

I am a strong advocate of prostatic massage for the symptoms of chronic prostatitis, and many of my colleagues agree with me, but there are some urologists who feel that regular sexual activity leading to ejaculation is the only way to empty the prostate of fluid. I do not fully agree with them, although I do agree ejaculation is very helpful in the treatment of congestive prostatitis, which is discussed in the next chapter. I do believe that regular sexual activity is an excellent urological as well as general physical and psychological prescription for all human beings, but I do not think it is the *only* prescription for a prostate that needs to be drained.

4

PROSTATITIS: CONGESTIVE AND IRRITATIVE

When a patient comes to see me with complaints of lower-back pain, a burning feeling in his penis during urination, urinary urgency or frequency, discomfort or pain after ejaculation, or hematospermia (slight bleeding with ejaculation), I am highly suspicious that his problems are related to the prostate. Often he has seen his general physician, who has ruled out other medical problems and, during a rectal examination, has noted that the prostate does not seem enlarged or have any hard nodules but does seem soft and boggy, filled with prostatic fluid. The symptoms the patient presents, as well as the reported findings of the referring doctor, lead me to suspect that the patient is suffering from prostatitis. If there are no reported instances of fever, chills, or other signs of malaise, I can usually rule out acute infectious prostatitis, but I cannot tell if the patient is suffering from congestive prostatitis or irritative prostatitis. Infectious forms can usually be ruled out by laboratory tests as well as by examination, as described in Chapter 3, although occasionally a viral or bacterial infection may not reveal itself in cultures and under the microscope.

I am then left with a very strong hunch, if not a definitive answer, as to the nature of the prostatitis from which the patient is suffering. Most often, a full and careful medical, social, and sexual history will give me the answer.

RANGE OF CAUSES

Patients suffering from congestive prostatitis—or, as it is frequently known, prostitosis—can be as different from one another as the nineteen-year-old motorcyclist with a girl in every section of town is from the aging pious priest deeply committed to his vow of celibacy. Diverse as they are, these men have one thing in common: each may be placing undue stress on his prostate.

Each day the normal prostate of a healthy man secretes about one-tenth to four-tenths of a teaspoon of prostatic fluid. This small amount is readily passed off with his urine. When sexually aroused, a man's production of fluid goes up four to ten times that amount, providing sufficient semen to carry the sperm cells through the urethra and expel them at the man's sexual climax. When arousal is not followed by ejaculation, the fluid manufactured to meet that demand remains in the prostate—though some of this fluid may be expelled if a man has frequent nocturnal emissions. If this fluid continues to accumulate in the prostate, the congestion it causes in the prostate can bring a man to a point of discomfort and lead to one or more of the symptoms I have described.

Most of the many men who suffer from congestive prostatitis find that their sexual habits are at the root of the problem. In cases where this is not so, the urologist must be alert to other possible explanations. For example, some men seem to produce more than the usual amount of prostatic fluid and fail to ejaculate all of it at climax. For such a man, treatment may have to be on a trial-and-error basis, but generally he can be afforded some relief. Some men suffer the symptoms of prostatic congestion—particularly a sense of pelvic heaviness or pain—but the examination shows no signs of congestion, and other studies reveal no urological problem. If they come away with a clean bill of health, such patients tend to become "doctor shoppers," looking for a surgeon who is willing to do exploratory surgery in search of some abnormality that might be causing the symptoms. Usually the surgery reveals nothing.

When I am confronted with such a case—symptoms of prostatic congestion with no physical evidence—I begin to look for underlying psychological reasons. Great anxiety about job, family, or school—not just about sex—can result in such symptoms. Sometimes I ask a few questions that allow the man to discuss his life more fully. Just my listening carefully and reassuring him that his symptoms will cease is sometimes enough to give relief. If his symptoms are not relieved, I usually refer him to a psychiatrist, psychologist, social worker, or minister for counseling. But it is bad policy to rush a patient off for emotional counseling until all bodily symptoms have been fully investigated by a physician. Sometimes a condition benefits from a combination of physical *and* emotional treatment. For this reason I work closely with all the helping professions and refer patients to many of them. Conversely, a social worker or psychologist might refer a patient to me because the patient has revealed problems with sexuality that indicate a potential urological problem. For example, a man might complain to his psychologist that often when he is talking to a pretty woman at a cocktail party, he has to excuse himself to go to the bathroom and urinate. He may simply be manifesting an anxiety about talking to a woman. But the wise psychologist knows that the patient may actually be suffering from prostatitis. Only when his frequent need to urinate interferes with pleasurable experiences does he become aware that he seems to have a urological problem. A urologist can clarify the matter. Such a case emphasizes why a urologist should take a full history and why a patient should be as honest and detailed as possible in giving the history.

Some urologists claim that men who present themselves with the symptoms described at the start of this chapter and who show no evidence of infection are simply the victims of unhealthy sexual practices. But such a label is too broad, and it reflects a rather narrow attitude.

It is not my wish to impose my own sexual preferences, beliefs, standards, or morals on my patients. Still, at times, I do believe that certain sexual practices can create prostatic problems for some people.

Following are descriptions of some of my patients, their habits, and the treatments I suggested for their complaints. Of course, where the treatment is controversial I will acknowledge that fact, in all fairness to both my readers and my highly respected colleagues.

VARIED SEXUAL ACTIVITY

Herbert was a fifty-four-year-old attorney in good general health who enjoyed a twice-weekly game of squash at his local club. He drank moderately and watched his weight carefully. His wife of twenty-five years was recovering from a hysterectomy after months of serious gynecological problems. Until her illness, they had had an active sexual relationship. As Herb put it rather wistfully, "I always was pleased to know I spent more time making love to my wife in a week than I did playing squash, but it's certainly not that way anymore." In the months prior to surgery, they had had sexual relations only occasionally, and she was still not feeling well enough for sex at the time he came to see me.

Herbert was suffering from some of the same symptoms as his older brother, who had recently had surgery for benign prostatic hypertrophy. He assumed that he was developing the same condition, so he came to see me. Upon examination, I was able to assure him that was not the case at all, but that his prostate was soft and boggy, and clearly congested. Because there was no infection, I was able to give him a prostatic massage on his first visit, and he was pleasantly surprised to find that he was almost immediately relieved.

I explained to Herb that, in my opinion, a prostate becomes "programmed" for a certain sexual pace. So when Herb abruptly changed his pace, his prostate wasn't prepared for the change. It continued to produce far more fluid than he could use. The result was painful congestion. Some researchers dispute this theory, but there is plenty of evidence to support my belief, so I am constantly alert to histories that reflect altered sexual patterns.

PROSTATIC MASSAGE

For Herb there were several possibilities. He could, of course, find himself a new and willing partner. He could ask his wife to help him ejaculate by manual or oral means, he could masturbate, or he could continue to see me or his family doctor for prostatic massage. It was clear that Herb, devoted as he was to his wife, would not consider seeking any other sex partner; such a suggestion from me would have been highly inappropriate. I told him that regular ejaculation would be helpful (one massage had drained his now congested prostate), but that the means to achieve this were up to Herb. He chose to come in regularly for prostatic massage, and he quickly felt much better.

Although masturbation might have been helpful, and I certainly have no objection to it on any ethical or moral grounds, I am not comfortable in recommending it to my patients. Perhaps this discomfort developed from my early years of urological experience when I would often see a teenage boy or man who had consulted me because of mild bleeding with ejaculation, irritation of the penis, burning on urination, and other such problems. These men usually had a common history; they all masturbated frequently; some did it three or four times a day. Thus, I came to believe that excessive masturbation was some-how involved in their problems. There seemed to be no other explanation.

In more recent times, I have seen young men with the same symptoms but a different history. They have inter-course several times a day, sometimes spending almost an entire night so engaged. Those young men who report that they delay ejaculation in order to satisfy their part-ner seem to get into difficulties with the above symptoms even more frequently than other young men.

So, undoubtedly, over my more than sixty years of urological practice, the large number of young men I have seen who reported a history of masturbation may have often stopped before ejaculation, then slowly started again, in order to make the experience lengthier and more exciting. They may have done this over and over again, until finally allowing themselves to climax.

In my opinion, and in the opinion of many other urologists, delaying ejaculation during either masturba-tion or intercourse tampers with the normal body rhythm and can lead to irritative prostatitis. For this reason, I am concerned by excessive masturbation or intercourse.

WHAT IS EXCESSIVE?

What do I mean by "excessive"? One friend of mine, a psychiatrist, used to define excessive as more than he thinks is ideal. He would define insufficient as anything less than he thinks is ideal. I define excessive masturbation or intercourse as more than the prostate can handle. If a man is getting into difficulties for this reason, it is excessive for him.

Dr. William Masters, who with Virginia Johnson directs the Reproductive Biology Research Foundation in St. Louis, has said publicly, and in direct answer to my coauthor's query, that masturbation never causes any problems. He also feels that manipulation of the penis to ejaculation, including the starting and stopping described above (it is called a teasing technique) is harmless. Dr. Masters stated clearly to my coauthor that he does not believe this teasing can lead to prostatic problems. Masters and Johnson have observed both heterosexuals and homosexuals in their St. Louis laboratories, and their findings regarding all areas of sexual functioning certainly are impressive. I shall not argue with these findings. But I shall continue to consider each patient as an individual and to try to prescribe the treatment that I think best suits my patient's physical condition and his psychological needs.

One Monday morning, a good-looking high school senior named Robert came to see me. He complained of severe pain in the pelvic area, which he had first noticed on the previous Sunday morning. I examined him and found nothing wrong except a rather congested prostate.

I suspected the reason for the problem. I have seen many Roberts in my office. And often on Monday mornings. Their stories are all strikingly similar.

This young man had been going steady with a lovely young girl whose ambitions were similar to his—to enter a good college and someday enter government or law. They usually spent Saturday evenings at her house, or if she were babysitting, he joined her on the job. They talked, watched some television, and got a bit romantic.

At his age, it is natural that Robert gets sexually excited quite easily. The same is true of the girl. Because they do not usually allow their kissing and lovemaking to progress to a point where she is almost orgasmic, she does not feel uncomfortable. But Robert, like most young men, quickly arrives at the brink of orgasm. This couple's moral standards prevent Robert's arousal from being relieved by permitting him an ejaculation. Later, at home, Robert takes a cold shower and goes to sleep. (A warm bath would probably be better; it might relieve him of some of the congestion he feels in his prostate.) When he wakes up the next morning, Robert's testicles are painful and swollen.

Robert has come to me for help and answers, like hundreds of Roberts before him. I prescribe rest, an anti-inflammatory drug, and application of an ice bag to the testicles. I also tell him to elevate his testicles by placing a towel under them. The real difficulty comes in advising him on how to prevent this problem from arising next Sunday and the Sunday after that. I do not feel it is appropriate for me to suggest that he and his girlfriend widen their relationship to provide him with an ejaculatory experience.

Most of my colleagues would suggest that this young man relieve his discomfort by masturbating when he gets home on Saturday night. It certainly is a logical solution.

But when I see young men like Robert, I try to explore their feelings as well as to explain to them what caused the problem. Often the patient himself will suggest the "prescription," if I am careful to listen. And sometimes the patient needs time to think about it. It is important for him to understand the cause of the problem, to be aware of alternative treatment plans, and to decide on one that is comfortable for him. Some people don't need direction; they simply need "permission" to do what they wish to do. I try to relate to them in a way that is accepting and nonjudgmental. I want to leave the door open for continued consultation if necessary.

Sometime after I treated Robert, he sent a classmate to see me. Tall, blond, and handsome, Larry was captain of the tennis team, a member of the school chorus, and popular with all his classmates. He was a smiling, confident young fellow who would make any parent proud. After a moment or two in my office, he confessed that he was scared. He had noticed some blood in his ejaculatory fluid, and he had a burning sensation when he urinated. He was sure he had picked up venereal disease and wanted me to check him out. All the tests were negative.

I had a hunch about what was causing the trouble, because Larry impressed me as a fellow who probably overdoes things a bit. I was right. Larry was dating Wynn, a girl who played on the tennis team with him. On the weekend before he consulted me, her parents had had to go out of town, but she had stayed home to play a tennis match. They had spent the weekend together. Larry reported to me that he had climaxed three times Friday night, three times on Saturday morning, then four times on Sunday. He was rather proud of his scorecard. He seemed disappointed when I didn't praise him for his sexual prowess. I think he expected me, as a urologist, to

41

be something of a sexual activities coach, who would urge him on to greater and greater achievements. I was sorry I didn't fit the image he had created. Instead it was my duty to explain to Larry that the prostate can't be suddenly expected to work overtime efficiently, after being virtually idle or working only a half-time schedule. I asked Larry what would happen if he got out on the courts for five sets of tennis after a long abstinence from the sport. He said he wouldn't be surprised if he developed a charley horse, and blisters all over his hand from gripping the racquet. Well then, I asked, could he see why his prostate, unprepared to produce the amount of fluid needed for several ejaculations, was signaling its fatigue and discomfort?

I didn't really have to suggest to Larry that he limit his sexual activity or, at least, pace himself more evenly. He came to that conclusion himself. Before Larry left, I did suggest he have a talk with Wynn. If this much sexual activity were unusual for her, she might also be suffering from a common genital disorder, "honeymoon cystitis," a bladder infection named in the days when most young women had their first sexual experiences on their honeymoon. Young women are highly susceptible to these bladder infections because their vaginal opening is often small and the penile thrusting during intercourse (particularly with the man on top) will be along the roof of the vagina, which is actually the first floor of the urethra and bladder. Bacteria present in the vagina are easily pushed into the urethra and bladder this way. Within a few days, these women may be acutely miserable with a bladder infection marked by frequent, burning urination and, occasionally, some blood in the urine. If these symptoms were present, I suggested Wynn speak to a gynecologist or to me.

FEAST OR FAMINE

Alan was a captain in the Merchant Marines. He came into my office with the all-too-familiar symptoms of prostatitis. He was a ruddy-faced, thirty-five-year-old man in good health, with no evidence of any genital bacteria or structural abnormalities. But he said his symptoms had persisted, on and off, for the last year. The pain in his rectal area was becoming more intense, and that was why he came to see me. He suspected cancer because he had seen some television commercials warning about it and recommending that all men have rectal examinations. I soon assured Alan that there was no evidence of any malignancy, but that his prostate was soft and boggy, and was probably congested. Alan's occupation gave me the clue to his problem. His sexual activity was "feast or famine," and this habit was playing havoc with his prostate's programming.

When he was at home, Alan and his wife had an intense period of sexual activity. He adored his wife and she adored him, so he was not the "girl in every port" type of seaman. When he returned to the ship, he was happy in his memories and sexually satisfied. He had no further sexual activity until he returned home. The feast on shore and the famine at sea were too much for his prostate. It would continue to produce more fluid than Alan could use at sea, so the fluid would accumulate and the prostate become congested. I was able to relieve Alan's congestion while he was in New York, but that wasn't much help to him while he was on duty. Alan might have looked for some other sexual outlets—extra-marital sex or masturbation—but he was not interested in either option, though friends had suggested those possibilities. The best I could do was to come up with a list of

43

reputable urologists in each of his regular ports so he could go to them for prostatic massage.

Many urologists consider massage of the prostate a poor substitute for intercourse as a means of emptying the prostate. I agree. Humans are sexual beings, not intended to use prostatic massage as a means of relief for their erotic tendencies. However, prostatic massage does empty the prostate when it has become painfully congested. It may well be the *only* way to empty it thoroughly so the man can enjoy sexual relations. Once the symptoms have been eliminated, there is no question that regular, satisfying sexual activity (ending in ejaculation) is just the thing to keep the urologist away, at least where congested prostatitis is concerned.

Nothing in John's sexual history indicated a reason for the clear case of congestive prostatitis he presented upon examination. Age forty-two, he was married to a woman of the same age, and they had a regular, fulfilling sexual relationship. The possible cause of John's problem came to light when he told me that he was a bus driver. Urologists have long noted that men whose occupations expose them to chronic vibration are prone to developing congestive prostatitis. Though the vibration may not be experienced by the patient as sexually stimulating, it *is* perceived by the prostate that way! So the prostate secretes fluid in keeping with its normal function. Because this fluid is not always expelled as quickly as it accumulates (even if the man is sexually active), the prostate tends to become congested. Truck drivers, motorcycle policemen, tractor drivers, and railroad workers are among the men whose jobs predispose them to this condition.

In Frank's case, tests showed that he was not suffering from infectious prostatitis, but he did have the symptoms of some prostate trouble. His social and medical history gave me a hunch about what the cause might be. He came from a large family, and he and his wife, both age thirty-five, had five youngsters of their own. Five were enough, Frank said, but he and his wife were reluctant to use any type of contraceptive device. So after their kindergartner had been born, they had begun relying on coitus interruptus—the interruption of sexual intercourse by withdrawing the penis from the vagina before ejaculation—to limit the size of their family. It is the most widely used method of birth control in the world, because is requires no advance planning, medical supervision, or costs. It is also one of the most unreliable methods, because prior to ejaculation a man often dribbles some semen containing enough sperm to impregnate a fertile woman. And it is *not* cost-free. It is expensive in terms of emotional and physical satisfaction and lack of reliability.

The man's preoccupation about withdrawing before he ejaculates places him in what Masters and Johnson call "the spectator role." He cannot lose himself in his and his partner's sexuality; instead he stands apart, psychologically speaking, watching to be sure he withdraws in time. As a pattern of sexual behavior, coitus interruptus is also undesirable because it can indeed cause prostatic congestion and irritation. It disrupts the normal body rhythm and may even diminish the volume of ejaculation. Certainly it diminishes the pleasure of the experience and, although there is no universal agreement on this subject, many urologists believe as I do that coitus interruptus is a common factor in prostatic problems.

When I explained this to Frank—and his wife, who joined us in the consultation room—he was troubled. He admitted that he had not been happy with this form of birth control, but he was in a quandary about what else to do. Frank and Catherine came to see me many years ago,

45

at a time when the Catholic Church was far less flexible than it is today, and when the pill had just come into use. They decided to speak with Catherine's gynecologist about a modified rhythm plan. They felt that since they liked frequent and regular sex, they might be able to rely on the coitus interruptus method only on those days the wife believed she was fertile. I saw Frank from time to time after that, and so far the method was working for them. No more pregnancies, no severe prostatic problems, *and* he and his wife were happy. These days I see far fewer patients who practice coitus interruptus for contraception, but occasionally I do see a man whose wife wishes him to withdraw before ejaculation. I have referred such couples for counseling, because generally they have other problems, both in and out of the marriage bed.

DIFFERENT TIMETABLES

Jim and his wife, Jane, are on a slightly different sexual "timetable," as many couples are. Jim is ready to climax about ten minutes after he has begun sexual intercourse, but his wife needs more time to reach orgasm. Both Jim and Jane take great pleasure in her pleasure. They had worked out a system in which Jim would hold back when he felt ready to ejaculate, so as to continue thrusting until his wife reached orgasm. This had been their pattern for many years, and it was satisfying for them. But this coitus prolongus, as it is called, led to irritation of Jim's prostate, and it kept him uncomfortable much of the time. The prescription: take warm sitz baths and allow ejaculation to occur spontaneously. If I had suggested only that, Jane would have remained unsatisfied and might eventually have ended up in a doctor's office complaining of pelvic congestion caused by constant stimulation that did not culminate in orgasm.

Here was a bright couple with no emotional problems. What they needed was sexual education, rather than marital or sexual therapy. At that time, the proliferation of books on sex had not yet occurred, and because they were neither experimental nor aware of the various alternatives for achieving sexual satisfaction, Jim and Jane had relied exclusively on sexual intercourse as the means for Jane to reach orgasm. I suggested to them that Jim might stimulate Jane orally and manually. They were very receptive and looked at my educational information as "permission" from an authority. Indeed it was. Not a prescription, since I would never prescribe sexual activities that might be unacceptable—merely permission.

When I talked with Jim a few months later, he reported a happier sex life for him and Jane than ever before, proving to me once again that some people simply need the opportunity to discuss problems with a knowledgeable physician in an unhurried atmosphere.

As demonstrated in the above cases, congestive and irritative prostatitis can have many causes, but the prognosis is good. A word of caution to anyone who might decide to live with the symptoms rather than change his sexual patterns: evidence indicates that congestive and irritative prostatitis make a man more susceptible to infectious prostatitis. And, as I said earlier, this can lead to chronic prostatitis, a highly treatable, but often incurable, condition. However—and this is important—neither infectious nor noninfectious prostatitis increases a man's chances of developing benign prostatic hypertrophy or cancer of the prostate. They are separate entities, and no studies have shown any relation among them.

5
ENLARGEMENT OF THE PROSTATE: BPH

Even a man who has avoided prostate trouble through most of his adult life is not safe from it when he reaches his retirement years. On the contrary, at this time of life, even the healthiest man is likely to develop prostate problems. Regardless of his identity—abstemious monk, traveling salesman, devoted husband, promiscuous sailor, or tractor-riding farmer—benign prostatic hypertrophy (BPH) is a strong possibility for a man of retirement age. BPH, the enlargement of the prostate gland, was nondiscriminatory long before the onset of equal opportunity legislation. Only one group of men *do* seem often to escape this condition: those who have been castrated (removal or shrinkage of testicles) through surgery or through intake of female hormones. For this reason, scientists believe that enlargement of the prostate gland is somehow related to the production and presence of male hormones.

The incidence of BPH in Asians had long been thought to be very low, but until recently, there were no studies that offered an explanation for this. Dr. George Nagamatsu, a prominent New York urologist of Japanese descent, long interested and familiar with this observation, discussed it with us. At one time, he and others did not know if the low incidence of BPH was genetically determined or related to Asian's low-cholesterol and low-meat diet. There are still no conclusive scientific studies, but recent evidence suggests that diet is an important contributory factor to the lowered incidence of BPH in those Asians who maintain their traditional diet. It had also been noted that the incidence of cancer of the prostate and the testes was low in Asians, but those Asians who no longer refrain from eating meat and fat appear to be at the same risk as Westerners.

Dr. Herbert Brendler, who has been chairman of the Department of Urology at Mt. Sinai Hospital in New York for many years, initiated an interesting collaborative study investigating the incidence of prostatic cancer in Asians, particularly Japanese. The study is continuing in cooperation with the Department of Urology at Keio University School of Medicine in Tokyo. Preliminary findings suggest that the incidence of prostatic cancer is significantly higher in Japan than previously reported. It is noted that when Japanese and other Asians live a nontraditional life-style in their native country, Hawaii, or the continental United States, the incidence of prostatic cancer increases, but still remains lower than that for the non-Asian population. Again, the genetic and environmental conditions that make this possible are not absolutely known, but there is clearly a suggestion that everyone would be healthier with less cholesterol and fats in his diet.

ENLARGEMENT ACCOMPANIES AGING

A man of sixty attending a class reunion would probably find that more than half of his former classmates had developed some enlargement of the prostate. By the time he is eighty, if he has not developed enlargement of the prostate, this man will be one of very few among his contemporaries who escaped it. That statement implies that BPH has reached "epidemic" proportions, which is not far from the truth. However, BPH is not an infectious condition, nor is it contagious. Despite its near universality in the elderly, it is not normal either, according to most experts.

Quite simply, BPH is an enlargement of the glandular tissue within the prostate capsule. Although it neither spreads nor attacks other tissues or cells in the body (which is why it is called benign, rather than malignant or cancerous), the enlargement of these tissues can push the prostate outward and narrow the urethra. As it presses against other structures, it can cause trouble, ranging from the minor discomfort of nocturia (waking up at night to urinate) to uremia or even renal failure (nonfunctioning kidney). Most men tend to ignore the first minor discomforts, but few go untreated to the point of almost complete kidney shutdown. The size of the enlargement does not always determine whether the patient will show symptoms, nor does the severity of symptoms determine whether the enlargement is a potential health risk. Because the degree of discomfort and pain is such a subjective thing and because symptoms tend to develop gradually, it is important to bring even the earliest symptoms, such as nocturia, to the attention of a doctor.

SYMPTOMS AND DIAGNOSIS OF BPH

The usual symptoms of BPH are similar to those of other prostatic disorders—hesitancy to begin urination, the slowness of the urinary stream, an urgent and frequent need to urinate, discomfort during intercourse or ejaculation, occasional blood in the urine or ejaculation, dribbling after urination, and—if there is kidney damage—

nausea, dizziness, or unusual sleepiness. The diagnosis is made easily when the examining physician finds the prostate soft, rubbery, and enlarged. An experienced urologist can often estimate even the size of the prostate from this examination. (The complete urological examination is described in detail in Chapter 2.)

The causes of BPH are basically unknown. But the effects vary, and so do the treatments. The physician considers the general health, age, and life-style of the patient. Often a man in his sixties tells me he expect diminishing health at his age and that he isn't ver optimistic about relief for his prostate condition. When tell him I was in medical school when he began kin dergarten and that I have continued to see patients and perform surgery long after my own prostate was r moved, he is usually surprised and encouraged. Son men get so involved in business and family life that th ignore the first symptoms of BPH and eventually suff such acute retention (inability to urinate at all) that th must enter the hospital on an emergency basis for rel and to avoid what could become a major medical em gency.

Paul was such a patient. The growth of the glan within his prostate was so slow that he was really aware of his symptoms. Oh yes, he needed to get u few times each night to urinate, but he expected tha sixty-three. He had just expanded his business, and oldest daughter had recently made him a grandfather the second time. With all his added responsibilities simply didn't take time for the usual checkup.

One wintry Saturday night, his family doctor ca me. He said that Paul's wife had just phoned to say Paul was in agony, suffering from acute retention. We him to the hospital and inserted a catheter into the p to drain the urine directly from the bladder. Paul's l

51

der contained over a *quart* of urine. He looked and fe
better within *minutes* after catheterization.

ACUTE RETENTION OF URINE

Sudden attacks of acute retention often follow exposure
to cold or consumption of alcohol, as well as the inges-
tion of cough mixtures that contain antihistamines, or
antihistamines alone. Doctors working in emergency
rooms in college towns will tell you that they often need
to treat a few of the "old grads" if the annual homecom-
ing game falls on a cold November Saturday. Paul's
attack was probably precipitated by a long afternoon
sitting on a cold park bench while he watched his grand-
son playing. With more regular checkups, his growing
prostate would have been spotted by his family physician, and he would have been sent to see me long before
this acute attack.

If I had examined Paul prior to this emergency, I might
have noticed that, in addition to BPH, he also suffered
from prostate congestion. I would have suggested regular prostatic massage. Some urologists feel that prostatic
massage is useless in treating BPH, but I have found that
massage can afford a great deal of relief, not only post-
poning surgery, but sometimes preventing it. Why? Because in so many cases, such as Paul's, the gland is
congested as well as overgrown, and the massage helps
to empty the gland of fluid. The symptoms we attribute to
BPH are often a result of the growth *plus* congestion. It is
difficult to assess which of these conditions is giving the
patient the symptoms, but since prostatic massage *can*
relieve the symptoms, it is extremely worthwhile to use
it. However—and this is important—the patient must be
watched carefully during this period to be certain that,

52

even though he is comfortable and without symptoms, no damage is occurring to his kidneys.

SURGERY FOR BPH

Of course, by the time I saw Paul, there was little question that he needed surgery. His prostate was not only quite enlarged, but it was also encroaching dangerously upon his urethra and preventing him from urinating. As soon as he was comfortable, and we had made sure that his general health was good and that he had no infection, we were able to operate, and he came through it well. In no time he was back to work and enjoying his family. The surgery I performed on Paul was a retropubic prostatectomy, one of the procedures described in detail in the next chapter.

Harry was an elderly man who was also referred to me only after an emergency occurred. He had been dribbling urine, both after urination and at other times during the day. He and his wife mistook this and his complaints of tiredness and weakness for normal aspects of aging— which they aren't—and neglected to report it to the family doctor. Except for these symptoms, Harry had been feeling quite well and had not been in touch with his family doctor for over a year.

The dribbling was due to benign enlargement of the prostate gland, and Harry's bladder was full of urine that he hadn't been able to void. He was suffering from what is called overflow incontinence, and some of this large amount of urine in the bladder was causing backflow pressure upon his kidneys. It was damaging the kidneys to such an extent that by the time Harry's wife reached the family physician, he was almost in a coma and had to be transported to the hospital by ambulance.

His wife explained that Harry had been extremely irritable, drowsy, and pale for the last few days, but she assumed he had just picked up a virus. There was no reason to admonish the distraught woman about waiting so long to consult a doctor. She was obviously feeling guilty as well as frightened. Fortunately for Harry and his wife, we were able to reverse the medical picture. We placed a catheter in his bladder, and by the next morning Harry was feeling much better. I operated a week later and removed a considerably enlarged prostate, and he made a satisfactory recovery.

Gerald was in many ways an "ideal" patient. He had just had his semiannual checkup with his family physician and, during the course of the history, had told his doctor that he was concerned because his urinary stream wasn't as strong as it had been before. He had noticed that in a public lavatory the stream no longer reached the back of the urinal. Sometimes, at home, urine would drip on the rim of the toilet bowl. He was a healthy man who had no other physical problems. His sex life hadn't changed, but this change in urinary pattern puzzled him enough so that he reported it to his doctor. That was a wise step because, even though his doctor routinely performed a rectal examination on all his patients over forty, he was particularly alerted to looking for some prostatic enlargement when he examined Gerald. His doctor felt some enlargement, but because it was not very large, he wanted it to be confirmed by a urologist and so sent Gerald to me.

I examined Gerald thoroughly and found some prostatic enlargement, and some mild congestion. There were no signs of infection. The x-rays confirmed my hunch, based on his symptoms, that there was some bladder outlet obstruction. However, tests also indicated that there was only a small amount of residual urine remaining in the bladder after he urinated and that there was no kidney involvement. He was not in any serious trouble with his prostate at this time.

If the prostate had continued to grow and the bladder outlet obstruction had become larger, the bladder would have had trouble emptying itself. Eventually, the bladder muscle might not have been able to keep pace with this obstruction, and it would just have "given-up." The result would have been a "decompensated bladder," one that can't empty itself. Urine remaining in the bladder not only causes many of the familiar prostatic symptoms, but it may also predispose a man to bladder infections. The collecting urine becomes increasingly stagnant and can serve as a perfect culture for growing bacteria. If this happens, the patient will begin to feel burning pain on urination, and often his urine will have a foul odor. Blood in the urine may also occur if the blood vessels in the bladder stretch so much that they suddenly rupture. Depending on the size of the vessel that ruptures, the blood may slightly color the urine, or it can be a frightening hemorrhage.

PROSTATIC MASSAGE

I explained all of this to Gerald, saying that he was in no danger of any serious trouble at this point, and that sometimes men go through a phase when their prostate bothers them, but then it causes no trouble for a long period of time, even without treatment. But I warned him that because there was evidence of major obstruction at the bladder outlet, he should report to me any additional symptoms. I particularly warned him to report immediately if he had any burning on urination, chills, or fever, which might indicate a urinary infection. And I told him to see his family physician regularly whether he had symptoms or not, and to come to my office twice a year so that I could see if any changes had occurred.

A few weeks later, Gerald called me to say that while he was still feeling fairly well, he had noticed some additional urinary symptoms, such as nocturia and urgency, and some pelvic heaviness. I suggested he come in, and I found that his prostate felt about the same size as it had before, but it now seemed slightly more congested. I massaged it, and the heaviness disappeared almost as soon as he was rid of the congesting fluid. I told him to see me or his family physician weekly for prostatic massage. The urinary symptoms lessened as well, and with this treatment he was able to avoid surgery for seven years. At that point, Gerald's prostate became much larger, his symptoms increased, and surgery was indicated. He had the simplest procedure, the transurethral resection (described in Chapter 6), and he was back to work in a few weeks.

For Gerald and other such patients, I find that prostatic massage is wonderfully therapeutic. In addition, I remind patients to avoid sitting too long in cold football stadiums, to limit their intake of alcohol and spicy foods, to avoid antihistamines, and to report any increased symptoms immediately.

Many patients who come to see me with the diagnosis of BPH ask me if anything in their past history could have caused this disorder. I assure them that sexual habits and infections appear to have no effect on the growth of the prostatic glandular tissue. At this time, no evidence shows that there is any way to avoid this growth, although it appears that the trace mineral zinc is somehow related to the health of the prostate. The value of taking supplementary zinc to prevent or to treat prostate problems has not yet been established. We will discuss it further in Chapter 8.

ALTERNATIVE TREATMENTS

The search still continues for a treatment—other than surgery—for benign prostatic hypertrophy. Doctors have known for a long time that castration will prevent BPH, but certainly no doctor would recommend it as a procedure for this purpose. It is also fairly well established that administering female hormones will diminish the condition, but the side effects of this treatment make it most undesirable for BPH. These female hormones have the same effect as surgical castration, in that they may reduce a man's libido (sexual desire), may cause some mild feminization, and may even render him impotent. Certainly this treatment is not preferable to surgery, so it is not common practice except for cancer of the prostate (described in Chapter 7). Occasionally some drugs are introduced for the purpose of reducing BPH, but as yet none have proved truly effective, and some that at first seem promising turn out to be disappointing.

Sometimes, even if the symptoms are mild and there is no kidney impairment, I will consider surgery because of the tremendous size of a prostate. As stated earlier, the average prostate weighs about 20 grams. When a prostate reaches a weight of about 40 grams, I usually recommend surgery. Some urologists disagree with me, preferring to wait until symptoms become more severe. Occasionally I see such massive enlargement of the prostate that I wonder how the patient has managed to void at all. In these cases, I know that it is just a matter of time before an emergency may occur, so surgery should surely be considered. Many cases of BPH are what I call "borderline." They could benefit from surgery, but they might also be controlled simply by massage and careful watching.

I always try to consider the life-style of the patient in these borderline cases. If there is no kidney impairment, and if the patient is afraid of surgery or has a personal reason to want to postpone surgery, I encourage him to give treatment a try. I explain that we can always operate later, if necessary. I know that some urologists make a firm policy of removing every prostate that is over a certain size, even if there are no meaningful symptoms and the x-ray study indicates that the patient is tolerating the prostatic enlargement well. I disagree because I have noticed, over my long practice, that many prostates grow so slowly that they never cause more than minor discomfort. If the patient doesn't mind living with the discomfort, why should I mind?

Most of my patients with BPH report that the condition does not alter their sexual activity, but some, unfortunately, are so concerned that they lose some desire. This problem will be discussed more fully in Chapter 9.

Among the many things I always explain to a patient with BPH is the fact that it is in *no* way related to cancer of the prostate. I explain to him that this growth is not cancerous, that it will not turn cancerous, and that it isn't the growth itself that will do damage to him but the fact that it may grow in such a way as to prevent urination.

This condition does not grant immunity to cancer of the prostate either. Benign prostatic hypertrophy and cancer of the prostate usually begin in different parts of the prostate and are unrelated. A man may have a benign prostatic hypertrophy that is treated either medically or surgically, and he can still develop cancer at some later date. Past bouts with prostatitis of the infectious, chronic, irritative, or congestive type will have no effect upon whether or not he develops BPH. However, any of these problems can coexist and, of course, such a condition makes both the symptoms and the treatment slightly more complicated.

For those patients who are either miserable with their symptoms or at risk of developing kidney impairment, surgery is clearly necessary. Except in some of the instances described above, there is usually no great urgency about surgery, so I try to schedule the operation when it is most convenient for all concerned. I try to prepare my patients for surgery so that they won't be needlessly frightened, and I find that most of them approach it in a rather positive fashion.

6
SURGERY FOR BENIGN PROSTATIC HYPERTROPHY

Surgery! Few men can face a prostate operation calmly. It doesn't matter whether this operation will be a man's first surgical experience or one of many. This operation is different; it involves basic masculinity.

The urologist who has determined that surgery is indicated has probably explained that there's no great rush, meaning that it isn't an emergency situation. But the operation cannot be postponed indefinitely. With time, the symptoms will probably worsen to a critical point.

Some patients are apprehensive, remembering the prostate operation their fathers had. It was a two-stage procedure generations ago, and the average hospital stay ranged from six to twelve weeks. (Today the two-stage operation—discussed later in this chapter—is seldom necessary, and when it is, it is a far simpler procedure.) I always try to explain to my patient just what I'm planning to do because many people either have no idea of what to expect or assume that their operation will be similar to the one some friend has had. Theirs may be quite different.

There are four kinds of surgical procedures that can be used to remove all or part of the prostate gland, and the surgeon chooses the procedure after considering many factors.

TUR (TRANSURETHRAL RESECTION)

If the prostate is not exceedingly large, usually I perform a TUR (transurethral resection). In this procedure, the doctor usually is able to remove most of the prostate gland from the capsule. Sometimes only part of the gland is removed, affording the patient relief from his symptoms.

In a TUR, an instrument is inserted into the penis and through the urethra (in the same manner as a cystoscope). Because no incision is made, a TUR is referred to as a closed operation. There are no telltale scars afterward to indicate that the man has had surgery. This is the preferred procedure for most urologists, except when the prostate is so enlarged that greater removal is necessary.

Sometimes I elect to do a TUR even in the case of a very enlarged prostate, if the man is elderly and his health is generally poor. Rather than subject him to open surgery, if I feel I can keep him comfortable for several years by merely removing a portion of the gland, I find this simpler method is best. Of course, I realize that if this patient's prostate is significantly enlarged, he may have trouble again in five or six years, and the procedure will then have to be repeated. Thus, before deciding which procedure is best for a patient, I must consider many factors: his age, general health, size of prostatic enlargement, and severity of symptoms.

Sometimes a urologist may base his choice of procedure on his own preference or area of expertise. A well-trained urologist is certainly entitled to a preference, but he should be able to do every one of the procedures well and, in my opinion, should base his choice of method solely on what is best for the patient.

The TUR involves the introduction of an instrument

into the penis, urethra, and bladder, and the removal of prostatic tissue by an electric cutting current. I usually explain to my patients that I'm simply widening a tunnel in the prostate. By doing so, I enlarge the canal through which the patient urinates, and this alleviates the discomfort he has been suffering. When the urethral glands within the prostatic capsule become enlarged, the prostate is pushed outward toward the urethra. This pressure causes an obstruction, which then creates the symptoms, urinary and otherwise, that the patient describes to his doctor. Most patients are surprised to learn that the symptoms are the same whether the enlargement is great or slight. It is up to the urologist to determine the extent of the enlargement and to decide whether surgery is required and, if so, what type to perform.

The first step of the TUR procedure is the insertion into the penis of a nonflexible metal sheath or a hard synthetic hollow tube. Through this tube is passed the sophisticated transurethral fiber optic microlens system, more commonly known as a resectoscope. One of the functions of this system is to show the obstruction clearly. The field is so completely illuminated with the fiber optic microlens system that a surgeon can see inside of the bladder as clearly as you might see a night ball game.

The urologist can then cut away tissue with an electric loop that is slipped through the hollow tube. He moves the loop back and forth and cuts away prostatic tissue, using it just as one would an electric knife in the kitchen. A foot pedal activates the electrical power, leaving his hands free for· the surgery. As he works, the surgeon constantly observes the entire area through a lens located just outside the penis.

Some urologists find that they can remove the same amount of tissue as would be removed through an incision. However, many reserve this procedure for cases in which relatively small areas of the prostate gland are to be removed.

Throughout the operation, the surgeon must be able to control internal bleeding, and he is marvelously equipped to do so. When he sees blood spurting from a vessel, he puts the loop right over the bleeding area and steps on the coagulating pedal of the maching to seal off the blood vessel. All hospitals have this sophisticated machine or system in their operating rooms. It has two pedals, one for cutting and one for coagulating.

When enough of the prostatic tissue has been removed to provide a good urinary canal and the surgical capsule (the shell) has been exposed, a catheter is inserted. This thin, smooth, flexible hollow tube, made of rubber or plastic, is put through the penis and the urethra, into the bladder. Its usual purpose is to draw urine directly from the bladder in cases where a patient can't or shouldn't urinate naturally.

HOSPITAL RECOVERY

The catheter I insert after a TUR—as do many surgeons—is a three-way catheter. This catheter has three openings. One allows fluid to go in, and one allows fluid to come out. The third has an inflatable balloon at the end which keeps the catheter from falling out. Through it I connect a stream of saline solution (water and salt), which helps to irrigate or cleanse the bladder. I usually use this saline solution for about twenty-four hours and then leave the catheter in the bladder merely to drain urine. I always remind the patient to drink plenty of fluids as a natural way to flush and cleanse his system.

In about four of five days, I can usually remove the

catheter, and the patient finds that he can urinate comfortably himself. A few days afterward, he can go home. There is no need to worry that removal of the catheter will be painful. When the balloon of the catheter is deflated, the catheter will simply slide out by itself if the patient stands up.

Occasionally a patient is unable to urinate comfortably on his own. It may be that he is just taking a little longer to heal than expected, or he may simply be frightened about trying to urinate. Many people, regardless of the kind of surgery they have, are afraid to urinate or to move their bowels after surgery. My reassurance to them that they are not alone in experiencing this anxiety is often all they need to take this next step toward independence.

I reinsert the catheter in the patient for whom urinating remains a problem. He is likely to be afraid this will hurt, remembering that it was initially inserted while he was anesthetized during surgery. I explain that it will be painless because I instill a local anesthetic preparation like Xylocaine into the urethra through the penis to eliminate any discomfort. (If your doctor should try to insert a catheter without medication, you have every right to resist.)

For the most part, a patient will feel fairly well about a week after a TUR. He will be out of bed within twenty-four hours after surgery, and for the first week or two he may have some slight burning or discomfort when he urinates, but this can be easily controlled with medication.

The patient who has done well and goes home within the average seven or eight days will usually find that he can get back to his normal routine fairly quickly. If his job is a fairly light one, in which he sits at a desk most of the time, he can get back to work about fourteen days after surgery. If he's a salesman who must be on his feet a lot, he will be more comfortable if he waits a little longer.

Someone who does moderately heavy work—a truck driver, for example—should plan on being away from the job for about three weeks, and a man who does very heavy labor should allow himself a month before returning to work. Of course, age and condition previous to surgery, as well as individual recuperative abilities, may alter this timetable.

SEXUAL ACTIVITY AFTER SURGERY

Regardless of how well he is feeling, I usually advise a man to abstain from sexual activity for at least a month after the operation. There is the possibility that slight bleeding may occur following the congestion that results during sex. I suggest to the man that he not place himself in situations where he is likely to become sexually aroused. It may just be a matter of having an open discussion with his partner or of putting aside his copies of *Playboy* for the month. Of course, I can give medication if the patient does get an erection and releases a little blood. Most patients find that they can comfortably wait a month to resume sexual activity and know that it will probably be as good as it was prior to surgery; it may in fact be more comfortable.

When the patient is discharged from the hospital after a TUR, I give him a prescription for a urinary antiseptic to prevent any possible infection or inflammation, and I tell him to take hot sitz baths rather than showers. If all goes well and he has no complaints, I ask him to see me in my office in about a week. However, I make it clear that if he develops any pain or bleeding or has trouble urinating, he should contact me or my associate immediately. I usually see a patient every few months after his first postsurgical visit; later, in about six months, I usually do an intravenous pyelogram in my office (as I did on his first visit) and suggest he see me every six months for a few years.

Many urologists prefer to do a TUR on even very large prostates. Interestingly, these doctors tend to cluster in certain parts of the country, and they will tell you that patients there don't want an incision because of the scar and that the patients insist on a TUR. I find that a little hard to believe. Though I know that patients today are more aware of their role as medical consumers than they once were, they seldom try to tell a doctor what kind of surgery he should perform—if they really have confidence in the doctor. (Patients who don't have confidence in their surgeon should respect this feeling and find a surgeon in whom they *do* have confidence.)

If a doctor tells a patient that he performs *only* TURs, I think that patient should find himself another doctor. Some of my colleagues tell me I'm being a little unfair to those surgeons who have refined the art of TUR to the extent that they can remove every last bit of a prostate gland this way (except, of course, the capsule, which is usually removed only in the case of cancer, to be discussed in Chapter 7), but I still hold to my opinion.

In the late 1920s and early 1930s, urology did not have the status of a specialty at the famed Mayo Clinic in Minnesota. Prostatectomy came under the heading of general surgery, because Drs. Charles and William Mayo refused to permit a department of urology. At that time, my friend and urological colleague, Dr. H. Carey Bumpus, was on staff at the Mayo Clinic. Dr. Bumpus was internationally famous for removing prostates instrumentally by transurethral resection. The reason he hadn't become adept at open surgical removal of the prostate was because the Mayos refused to allow the doctors in the urology department to perform any open surgery.

The Mayos decided that a grade-1 or grade-2 prostate (grading was determined by the size of prostate enlargement) could be operated upon by the men who could use the transurethral instruments—that is, the urologists. Grades 3 and 4 (the larger prostate) had to be turned over to the general surgeons. Dr. Bumpus told me that when he, as a urologist, did the examination and evaluation of patients, he never found anything larger than grade two! In that way, the urologists ended up operating on all the patients with BPH. When Dr. Bumpus worked with me in New York City in the early 1930s, he learned to do open surgery, as most of us in the East were already doing.

However, he did remove giant prostates transurethally, and I suspect that, today, those urologists who perform only TURs were trained by older urologists who worked in surgical departments where they were permitted to use only this procedure.

I feel that if a man's prostate is so enlarged that I can't easily remove the entire gland by a TUR within one hour, I would rather perform open surgery. If the patient is in his sixties and is in fairly good health, and his prostate is large, chances are good that he will be back in five or ten years with the same symptoms if I perform an incomplete TUR. He will be older, perhaps not as healthy, and he will need another surgical procedure. This potential problem can be avoided if I remove the entire prostate gland the first time, either by TUR or by open surgery. In an older man, I sometimes compromise and do a partial TUR. This affords him comfort, and minimizes any risks.

To remove all of the prostate, all urologists are trained

to perform two procedures in addition to the TUR: the suprapubic and retropubic prostatectomies. Although some urologists prefer one to the other, I do both regularly.

SUPRAPUBIC PROSTATECTOMY

In the suprapubic prostatectomy, an incision is made through the skin below the navel and brought down to a point just above the pubis (the first bone below the navel) in the lower abdomen. Depending on the size of the individual, the incision is about four to six inches long. The incision is made through the skin and its lining, the fascia. The muscles covering the bladder are separated, and an incision is made into the bladder. The surgeon is then able to see if there are any stones, tumors, or diverticuli (outpouchings) in the bladder, all of which can easily be removed if necessary. The prostate, also clearly visible, is next removed.

All bleeding vessels are sutured, and these stitches dissolve by themselves after surgery. After all the bleeding is controlled, a catheter is passed through the penis into the bladder. This catheter is used for both irrigating and emptying the bladder. Just before the bladder is tightly closed by the surgeon, another (suprapubic) catheter is put in place. This one is inserted in the bladder, where it goes through the muscle fascia, and skin, and comes out just below the umbilicus, serving to keep the bladder empty of urine and irrigating fluid.

The continuous irrigation is discontinued in one to three days, and the suprapubic catheter is removed a few days later. The catheter that is in the penis remains in place for a week. Its purpose is just to remove urine from the bladder and to permit normal healing. When it is removed, on about the seventh day, the patient is usually able to urinate on his own. If he has trouble urinating, a catheter is reinserted after instilling a local anesthetic preparation, just as after a TUR.

RETROPUBIC PROSTATECTOMY

The same incision is made in a retropubic prostatectomy as in a suprapubic. The incision is made through the skin and the fascia, the muscle is separated, and all the intestines are pushed away from the bladder. Instead of opening the bladder, however, the incision is made into the prostatic capsule and the enlargement is then removed. After the prostate is removed, all bleeding vessels are sutured, and a three-way catheter is passed through the penis, the capsule, and into the bladder. This three-way catheter is identical to the one used in a TUR. The balloon is inflated, the capsule is sutured closed, and the muscle, fascia, and skin are also tightly closed.

In this procedure, because the bladder is left closed, there is no need for drainage with the suprapubic catheter. All the draining and irrigation are done through the three-way catheter. This method takes about the same amount of time to execute as the suprapubic, but often it appears less stressful to the patient than a suprapubic procedure, presumably because the bladder is not cut and there is no tube in the bladder. Many urologists who use both methods find it difficult to explain why they prefer one or the other. The retropubic is a bit more difficult in obese patients because the doctor has to work in a small space. When I have an obese patient, my preference is a suprapubic prostatectomy, but with a thin or medium-built individual, I might choose to do a retropubic.

Urologists will consider several factors in deciding which procedure to use, based on their training and ability, and their personal familiarity with either procedure. I suppose I have instinctive feeling in each case as to which I plan to use, and I would say that my practice is about evenly divided between suprapubic and retropubic when open surgery is indicated rather than a TUR.

Whether the patient has had a suprapubic or retropubic prostatectomy, he can probably plan to go home somewhere between ten and twenty-one days after surgery. He can bathe, shower, and return to work shortly after that. Just as after a TUR, the man whose occupation requires heavy labor needs to wait a little longer to resume work than does the man whose job is sedentary. About a month after surgery, he can do anything he did before surgery. Including sex. I usually suggest that patients wait four to six weeks after surgery to resume sexual activity, but many of my patients don't listen to me and have intercourse three weeks after surgery without any side effects. I do not anticipate that my patients will have any problems with sex following surgery for BPH unless, of course, they had sexual problems prior to their prostate trouble. Chapter 9 will cover this topic more fully, along with the issue of fertility following surgery.

PERINEAL PROSTATECTOMY

There is another procedure called the perineal prostatectomy. In the New York area, where I was trained and have my practice, very few urologists regularly perform perineal prostatectomies. In this procedure, the incision is made through the perineum, the area between the anal opening and the scrotum, and the prostate is removed through that incision. This is a direct route to the prostate and may sound like a good idea, but it frequently leaves the patient with two unhappy side effects. Nerves are often severed, leaving the patient impotent, and very often stricture formation, something like scar tissue, occurs.

Stricture formation can follow any of the surgical procedures described, but it is much more frequent with the perineal approach. If there is stricture formation in the urethra, I usually dilate the patient in the office a few times to help relieve him of his discomfort in urinating. Dilation is done by inserting a thin metal instrument through the penis and urethra to stretch the urethra, and then removing it. Of course, just as I do before inserting a catheter or cystoscope, I instill some Xylocaine or other anesthetic to make the procedure painless. Without dilation, the patient will continue to suffer the same discomfort he felt prior to surgery.

It should be obvious that I am not at all in favor of the perineal approach for BPH. I believe that the other procedures serve much better for the purpose of removing the prostate gland. Some advocates of the perineal approach may say that in this method the physician can get a good view of the rear of the prostate, which is where cancer often exists, but that doesn't seem a satisfactory reason to me. Examination prior to surgery will most often inform the doctor if cancer is present or suspected. Laboratory tests (pathology report) on the tissue removed during a biopsy or surgery will confirm any such suspicion. Other proponents of the perineal approach may also argue that this procedure leaves little postoperative discomfort and that recovery is rapid, so that it is a good method for the older patient who doesn't really care if he is left impotent. Personally, I have rarely met a man of any age who was willing to be rendered

71

impotent, even if he wasn't sexually active at the time. For this reason, and because of the higher risk of stricture formation in the procedure, I abandoned its use long ago.

In some medical centers, urologists are attempting a new method of surgically treating BPH by cryosurgery. They insert a probe containing liquid nitrogen through the penis and urethra to the prostate, shrinking away swollen tissue. In New York, most of my colleagues with whom I have spoken are not enthusiastic about cryosurgery for BPH, but they do agree that it may have possibilities for the future, possibly in cancer of the prostate.

TWO-STAGE PROCEDURE

In the beginning of this chapter, I mentioned the two-stage procedure that doctors used to perform almost exclusively back in the early 1920s and 1930s. In that procedure, the first stage consisted of draining the bladder by making a four- to six-inch opening below the umbilicus. A tube was then placed in the bladder for drainage of urine. Anywhere between seven and fourteen days afterward, an incision was made through the skin, muscle, and bladder, and the prostate was removed. In those days, packing was placed in the prostatic cavity (the area from which the prostate had been removed), and then the bladder, muscle, and skin were closed around another drainage tube. In about two to five days, the packing was removed. Each of these three steps required general or spinal anesthesia. The patient remained in the hospital another few weeks.

This procedure is usually not necessary today, but it is still practiced if the patient has neglected treatment of simple surgery until he has reached the "end of the line" and has practically developed early uremia, with partially destroyed kidneys; or if the patient has such unrelated medical problems as cardiac or pulmonary conditions that may respond more favorably to this kind of procedure.

CYSTOSTOMY

The first stage of the modern procedure, known as a cystostomy—where the tube is first placed in the bladder as described above—is actually a rather simple procedure. Most patients remain in the hospital for about ten to fourteen days before the second stage is done, at which time the prostate is actually removed. Packing is no longer routinely placed in the prostatic cavity.

Sometimes I will send a patient home after ten days of drainage, and then he is brought back to the hospital anywhere up to nine months later for the second stage. During the period at home, the patient is not bedridden, nor is he limited in most of his activities. Many of these men go back to work. They can exercise by walking or playing golf; they can drive a car, travel, or do whatever they were normally able to do before surgery.

Improved technology has made the two-stage operation much easier than it was when I first trained in urology. The patient who is at home between stages of surgery wears a leg bag, which collects urine coming from the tube that is in the bladder. He can easily learn to care for the tube and bag himself, and he learns to remove it in order to take a tub bath or shower. After the second stage of the surgical procedure, when the prostate is actually removed, his recovery is usually very good; most men function even better than they did prior to surgery.

Obviously there is no particular operation that is perfect for everyone with BPH. Instead, the procedure chosen depends on a combination of such factors as the extent of prostatic enlargement and the patient's general health and age. The urologist's own particular preference will also be important, and it should be respected, provided he is willing and able to perform whichever procedure is appropriate to the case.

With the patients on whom I plan to perform a TUR, I always make a point of saying that it is possible—although very infrequent—that when the patient is in the operating room, I may have to decide on open surgery. If, for some technical reason, the necessary instrument cannot be inserted, I will not be able to do the TUR. It's difficult to say why the instrument won't go through, especially since the patient may have been successfully cystoscoped in my office only a week before. Sometimes the final decision to perform a TUR must await final inspection of the bladder with a cystoscope after the patient has been anesthetized, but before surgery begins. All urologists have had such an experience at one time or another. That's why I always tell a patient that if for some reason I can't do the TUR I am planning, I will do a one-stage suprapubic. I prepare my patient for this slim possibility beforehand because if he is expecting to have a TUR but wakes up with an incision, it can be a very frightening experience. Of course, after surgery I give him a full explanation of what happened.

PREPARATIONS FOR SURGERY

Regardless of the procedure planned, some presurgical preparations are the same for all patients. In most hospitals, certain routine tests are done, such as electrocardiogram, chest x-ray, and blood tests. The tests specific to the surgery—IVP, for example—have been done prior to the decision to bring the patient into the hospital—unless, of course, it is an emergency. These routine tests are often done at the time of admission even before the patient goes up to his room.

I never operate on a patient without a medical "go ahead" from his internist. As explained earlier, I insist on a thorough history from the referring physician, and if this is not available, I do much of it myself or send the patient to another internist.

After admission, and after surgery, regular hospital medical staff (the "house staff") will often take a history and examine the patient. This is standard procedure in all hospitals, and the patient's own doctor often relies on these doctors for progress reports between visits. However, if a patient has concern about any house staff procedure he should feel free to question it. He can at least make sure his doctor has ordered it or is aware of it.

In his room, prior to surgery for any of the described procedures, a man is shaved of his pubic, scrotal, and abdominal hair. This is usually done on the evening before or on the day of surgery.

Naturally, the type of anesthesia is an important consideration. I usually prefer spinal anesthesia for a TUR, suprapubic, or retropubic prostatectomy. For a two-stage suprapubic, I like to do the first stage with a local anesthetic (Xylocaine-like) injected into the skin below the umbilicus, and for the second stage I ask for general or spinal anesthetic. But I let the internist and anesthesiologist make the final decision.

Except in emergencies, I always insist that the anesthesiologist meet the patient the day before any surgery. It gives them an opportunity to discuss mutual concerns and make the best final decision regarding the type of anesthetic. Some patients want to be awake; others insist on being asleep. Accordingly, there is a choice of spinal (awake) or intravenous (asleep) anesthetic. The ether mask, which you may remember with dread if you had your tonsils removed as a child, is no longer used. Today most patients are made very groggy by injection before they even reach the operating room.

During any of the procedures for prostatectomy, there may be a need for blood transfusions. I always remind my patients that, unless they are a member of a blood program which offers them free blood replacement, they should consider asking family and friends to donate blood for them. Blood is expensive, and most insurance policies, Medicare included, do *not* pay for the first few pints. If the patient is in good health, and his medical doctor agrees, an even better idea is for him to donate his own blood in advance of the surgery. This is called autotransfusion. A person donates his own blood up to thirty-five days prior to surgery, and this blood is stored for use during or following surgery. Blood can be stored longer, but only if it is frozen. Freezing is expensive, and not all hospitals have the facilities to freeze blood. Gail Button, RN, of the Mount Sinai Medical Center Blood Bank says that the ideal time for the "donor-recipient" to come into the Blood Bank to be bled is three weeks prior to surgery. This enables the patient to fully recover from the donation, and allows the blood to remain fresh if needed during surgery or in the week following surgery. If the blood is not needed by the patient, it then becomes available for some other patient. Autotransfusion is a fine idea because it is healthier and safer than receiving blood from an unknown donor.

Surgery to correct other conditions is not usually performed at the same time as BPH, although certain conditions in the urinary tract might be handled simultaneously. If there is a diverticulum of the bladder (an outpouching), it can be removed when either a suprapubic or a retropubic is performed. If there are stones in the bladder, they can be removed, too.

After surgery the patient will no doubt be removed to a recovery room and then, in some hospitals, to a surgical intensive care unit. When his condition seems stable, he is moved back to his own room. The timetable for this varies widely, so family and friends should not worry about how soon the patient returns to his own room.

RECOVERY AT HOME

It has been my experience that by describing the planned procedures of a prostate operation to my patients, I can alleviate much of their presurgical fear. I also find that some of their apprehension is put to rest during the initial office visits when they discover that cystoscopy is not painful and that, likewise, having something inserted into the penis is not unbearable. Most patients are so miserable with their symptoms of BPH that they are really eager for relief. And relief is what they usually get, though some minor symptoms may persist temporarily until all healing takes place. For example, a man may still feel the urgent need to urinate frequently, and his urinary stream may still be weak. He *may* also have some urinary leakage, occasional bladder spasms, and some bleeding that causes a slight discoloration of urine. These symptoms are not inevitable, nor are they cause for panic. I always tell my patients to call me about any such concerns so that we can discuss it fully.

Most men experience a vast improvement. Being able to sleep through the night without hourly visits to the bathroom is enough to make any man look and feel younger. Sexual functioning is often improved, and life really can begin anew after the surgery. Within a few months, the prostate trouble seems like a distant memory. In fact, many of my patients would forget to come back for checkups if I didn't send them a reminder to do so!

7

CANCER OF THE PROSTATE

Even after more than sixty years of being a physician, I still get a heavy feeling in my heart when I have to tell a patient or his family that he has cancer, even though the outlook for cancer of the prostate is considerably brighter than it was years ago. Today I am often able to assure a man that he has every reason to expect a long and comfortable life. The general picture is steadily improving because better treatments are constantly being developed.

Most people shudder at hearing the word "cancer." To them it is synonymous with a slow and painful death. But that's not always the situation. Many people expect only the worst, but if they understood cancer better, they would know that often it can be treated successfully, and they would see why early detection is so very important.

Cancer, quite simply, is an uncontrolled growth of abnormal cells. These cells do not stay in one place; instead, they penetrate into surrounding tissues between normal cells, crowding them out. The cancerous cells form tumors and tend to spread through the blood or lymph systems to other parts of the body, where they create new tumors. Cancer cells can spread in an orderly fashion or in what seems to be in a chaotic way. A cancerous tumor that originates in one part of the body may show up almost immediately or much later in a

79

distant area. However, when cancer is discovered very early, while it is still contained in one place, it can often be treated successfully by surgery, radiation or drugs. Even if not absolutely cured, it may remain inactive or dormant for many years—perhaps for a lifetime. "Cure" is a word sometimes—if rarely—used by those who treat cancer when the cancer seems to have been completely eliminated. However, I am more comfortable with the phrases, "under complete control" or "no evidence of disease."

Cancer of the prostate is almost always a primary cancer—that is, one that originates in that site. It does not travel from other parts of the body to the prostate, although some cancers may travel to areas close to the prostate. The cancer begins its growth in one lobe of the prostate and, if untreated, will probably spread (metastasize) through and out of the prostate capsule and eventually through the lymph system to the bones, lungs, chest, and even brain. It is a treacherous as other cancers, but, if discovered early, highly treatable.

CAUSES AND INCIDENCE

Cancer of the prostate is so common that, according to reliable estimates, by age eighty almost all men have some beginnings of it. Even if the cancer is untreated, or treated very conservatively but carefully watched, most of these elderly men will never have symptoms of cancer, and will die of unrelated causes. Few men under forty ever have cancer of the prostate, but from the ages fifty-five to seventy-four, it becomes the third highest cause of cancer deaths in men, exceeded only by lung, colon and rectal cancer. After age seventy-five it becomes the second highest cause of cancer deaths in men, following lung cancer. Despite this high incidence, over-all, prostatic cancer only accounts for ten percent of cancer deaths in men, as compared to thirty-four percent caused by lung cancer. Because it is virtually only a disease of older men, it has been on the rise as an increasing number of men live long enough to develop the disease. When diagnosed early, however, it can have a good prognosis. Many patients whose prostate cancers I initially diagnosed ten to twenty-five years ago are still living full and healthy lives.

One of my greatest joys in practicing medicine oc-curred a few years ago when a man I had first treated many years previously for cancer of the prostate called me to say that he was planning to retire to Florida and wanted me to give him the name of a good urologist there. I had seen him regularly for twenty years, and there had been no sign of recurrence of the disease. He looked at me as a "miracle man" for "curing" him, but the truth is that he was an ideal patient who had seen his family physician regularly and was referred to me at the very first suspicion of cancer of the prostate. Most patients are neither so careful nor so lucky. Too often I don't get to see them until the cancer has invaded areas outside of the prostatic capsule.

The cause of cancer of the prostate is unknown. It is a disease found almost exclusively in humans—which, of course, prevents meaningful experiments in animals. There is no clear evidence that smoking, drinking, or any environmental factors have anything to do with the de-velopment of prostatic cancer. There does not seem to be any relationship between sexual activity and cancer of the prostate, although it does occur more frequently among married men than among single men. Incidence is also higher among blacks than among whites. Until re-cently the incidence was low in Asians or those of Asian extraction; the reasons for this discrepancy are not fully understood, although it may be both genetically and environmentally (diet, in particular) related. There seems to be no way to prevent the onset of cancer of the prostate, but some evidence shows that men with low-cholesterol diets, as well as those who are vegetarians or eat a great many green and yellow vegetables, have fewer cases of prostatic cancer.

IMPORTANCE OF EARLY DETECTION

Cancer of the prostate usually originates as one or several collections of malignant cells in the outer portion of the gland beneath the fibrous, or true, capsule. When the family physician who examines a patient rectally during his regular checkup feels a hard nodule, he will suspect cancer and quickly send you to a urologist for a more definitive diagnosis. A nodule is a stony, hard mass of any size, which might be cancer, but which might just be a stone in the prostate or nothing more than an inflammation. Often only the urologist can tell for sure.

Regular rectal examinations of the prostate are as vital for men as pap smears and breast examinations are for women. Unfortunately, radio, television, and magazines do not sufficiently emphasize this fact. There is no doubt in my mind that a good number of the estimated twenty thousand men who die every year in the United States from cancer of the prostate could be saved as a result of this simple examination.

Most people ask two basic questions on this subject: first, how does a doctor decide that it is cancer of the prostate? and, second, are there symptoms?

A diagnosis of prostatic cancer is reached in several ways: by rectal examination, by various blood tests, and

by examination of tissue from the prostate. Because the malignancy usually originates in the part of the prostate that does not cause urinary obstruction, there are seldom any of the obvious symptoms a man might experience in prostatitis or BPH. In general, by the time a man becomes aware of cancer-related symptoms, the cells have probably spread throughout the capsule.

If the cancer has spread beyond the capsule into lymph nodes or bones, there are other symptoms. Pain in the pelvis, lower back, or upper thighs are often those signs that first send a man to his physician. At this point, the cancer has probably spread beyond the capsule. Treatment may still be successful, but I cannot be as fully optimistic as when the cancer is discovered before it has spread.

After a routine operation for BPH, I often get a report from the pathologist showing some malignant cells in the gland. This cancer is at so early a stage that even the rectal examination by a highly trained and skilled urologist would not have revealed it. For such a patient, the outlook is extremely bright and, if he follows my recommendations, he should usually have no problems. But, before describing the various treatment plans for patients with cancer of the prostate, I would like to focus more specifically on the way in which I arrive at the diagnosis.

DIAGNOSTIC STEPS

The first thing I must do is to rule out the possibility of a stone in the prostate, or an inflammation, even though I may be highly suspicious that it is cancer. Therefore, I conduct my regular examination, as described earlier. If it does not seem to be a stone or an inflammation, I do a simple procedure called a transrectal biopsy, in which a

needle is inserted into the patient's rectum and enough of the tissue is aspirated through the needle to be examined by a pathologist. Many urologists do a biopsy of the prostate by removing tissue through the perineum. This procedure can be done on an outpatient basis, but I find that most patients prefer to enter the hospital for it. In addition, this allows me to conduct further tests for a more complete picture of the patient's general health and the extent of the prostatic cancer, *if* the biopsy proves it is cancer.

These studies help the doctor to decide on treatment and to establish a base line for the disease. The exact boundaries of the malignancy must be established when the patient is first diagnosed, or there is no way to determine if the treatment is helping him.

Blood tests show blood alkaline and acid phosphatase levels. An elevated acid phosphatase level suggests matastasis because acid phosphatase is an enzyme produced in the prostate gland, and its production increases with prostatic cancer, releasing more of it into the bloodstream. However, an increased level of this enzyme may occur for reasons other than the spread of cancer. For example, if a man has been examined rectally and the prostate has been massaged even slightly, acid phosphatase from it will travel into the bloodstream. Blood drawn from him within twenty-four hours will show an elevation of this enzyme that has no connection whatsoever to cancer of the prostate. Conversely, the disease may metastasize, yet not cause an elevated acid phosphatase level. Obviously, this test must be corroborated by other tests, but it does alert the doctor to a probable danger.

Radioimmunoassay, a relatively new analytical technique, can be used to measure substances present in the blood in amounts too small to be detected by other

methods. Thus, it can spot the most minute increase in the blood's acid phosphatase level at an earlier time than was possible with previous standard tests. Some physicians have suggested that it may eventually be used for mass screening of prostate cancer, just as the pap test is now used for early detection of cervical cancer in women. However, radioimmunoassay is unlikely to replace the digital rectal examination. Dr. Patrick Guinan, chairman of the Division of Urology at the University of Illinois School of Medicine in Chicago, demonstrated in a recent study that the digital rectal examination is still one of the best methods of detecting cancer of the prostate, despite all the tests available. As he explains, "Before 1920 it was the *only* way." Of course, when I learned my urology (I graduated medical school in 1919), it was indeed the only way, and so we learned it well, as did all physicians. I was happy to learn of Dr. Guinan's findings because it reassured me that the men and women who are enrolled in medical school today will continue to be well trained in this low-cost, easy-to-perform test that can be done anywhere and anytime.

In addition to the above, other tests can help the doctor detect any spread to distant organs. Bone x-rays, surveys, and scanning are useful; but here again, in x-ray examination, such other bone diseases as Paget's Disease (a generalized skeletal disease, in which bones may become thick and soft) may closely resemble cancer of the prostate that has spread to the bones.

Often the urologist will call in a hematologist to check a sample of bone marrow for suspected spread of cancer from the prostate to the bones, when it has not been absolutely confirmed by other tests. He might want to consult a medical oncologist, an internist specifically trained to treat tumors. The lymph nodes may also be x-rayed to determine if there has been a spread from the prostatic gland. Such tests help the urologist to determine the extent of the disease before he begins treatment, and to select the most appropriate treatment.

What happens if cancer of the prostate is allowed to go untreated? In some cases, it will be fatal because of the blockage it causes around the urethra, resulting in complete kidney shutdown, or because of its spread to other vital organs.

APPROPRIATE TREATMENTS

In some men over seventy, it is possible that a prostate cancer will not do any damage, even if left untreated, because this type of cancer grows very slowly in elderly men. However, I feel—as do many of my most esteemed colleagues—that it is risky to do nothing, just waiting to see if it will grow. Therefore, I usually suggest that the patient start taking very small doses of stilbestrol (a synthetic form of estrogen, a female hormone given in pill form), and I examine him at frequent intervals, keeping an eye on his acid phosphatase level. Usually, such a patient shows no advance of the disease. The effect of stilbestrol is to reduce the amount of testosterone, the male hormone, in a man. Since the prostate needs male hormones to grow, the testosterone reduction stops or retards the growth of the cancerous prostatic tissue.

In 1941, Dr. Charles Huggins introduced the concept of reducing male hormones to treat cancer of the prostate. By surgically removing the testicles, and giving the patient female hormones by mouth, he achieved some remarkable successes. I had the privilege of hearing him in Chicago at a meeting of the American Urological Association when he first described the treatment. Upon returning to New York, I was one of the first doctors there to perform this procedure, called a bilateral orchidectomy (removal of both testicles, leaving scrotal bag intact). Some of the patients I treated in the 1940s lived on for another generation and died of unrelated causes. Though doctors have come a long way in diagnosing and treating cancer of the prostate, many of the most eminent American urologists believe that the basic method introduced by Dr. Huggins is still the best.

Today, cancer of the prostate is described in definite stages agreed upon by almost all medical centers and urologists. However, the method of treatment varies, depending on many factors: the age and general health of the patient, the stage of the cancer, and the results of current research studies on prostate cancer. At this time, no single treatment for a specific stage of prostatic cancer has been proven best. Any well-trained, up-to-date urologist will be aware of all the accepted methods and will make his choice based on what he feels is right for his patient.

A pathology report may reveal only microscopic beginnings of cancer within the prostate gland, or the cancer may be localized within the capsule, consisting of only a small isolated nodule and causing absolutely no urinary symptoms. The cancer can also spread beyond the capsule to near or distant sites, including the bones. There may or may not be urinary symptoms.

HORMONAL TREATMENTS

Some very early stages of cancer will respond well to female hormones, called estrogens. These hormones are administered in the form of small pills, taken on a regular basis. They do produce some side effects, which I am always careful to explain to patients. Some time ago, cardiac conditions were noted to arise in many patients. It was a case of the "cure" being as bad, if not worse, than the disease! However, the risk of this effect is reduced considerably by giving much smaller amounts of stilbestrol, and studies show that smaller doses work against the cancer just as well.

There is the possibility that, in some men, these estrogens will lead to reduced libido and limit their ability to achieve erection. Even in small doses, the female hormone can cause some enlargement of a man's breasts (gynecomastia). To avoid this side effect, doctors can treat the breasts with small doses of radiation beforehand, usually three treatments of 300 rads each, a total of 900 rads to each breast.

The stilbestrol may cause some lessening of beard and some alteration of body shape. Men who are very thin and athletic-looking may develop a tendency to become fatter and thinner-skinned. Generally, these changes are hardly noticeable to anyone but the patient himself and can be minimized if he stays in good shape through proper diet and exercise.

These slightly feminizing effects occur because the female hormones atrophy (shrink) the testes and reduce the androgens (male hormones) in the body. These effects are similar to those achieved by removal of the testicles, and for this reason many men fear that they will be turned into eunuchs with high soprano voices. This circumstance is entirely different, for such eunuchs were castrated before puberty—a crucial difference. The genitals of the young boy have not attained full maturity, and he may not yet have developed an interest in sexual activity. But for the man who has had a full quota of male hormones throughout his life and has perceived himself—and been perceived by others—as a "complete" man, the results of a small dose of female hormones are negligible. Still, it is a matter that should be frankly and carefully discussed with a patient prior to treatment.

SURGICAL TREATMENT

For more advanced stages, various treatments are favored by individual urologists at medical centers throughout the world. When it is appropriate for a patient to have his testicles removed (orchidectomy), sometimes he can't bear to contemplate surgery. I tell him that, although he might lose some interest in sex and some ability to perform sexually, this effect is not certain. However, it *is* certain that if treatment is indicated, it would be foolish to ignore my recommendation. I explain to him that the removal of the testicles will not be apparent, since the scrotum remains, and that it can be filled with synthetic substance so it looks exactly the same. The patient will, however, become sterile. Although sexual intercourse may be normal, no pregnancy can result. For most of my patients, sterility is not a concern, for they are usually past the age in which they wish to become fathers.

Another surgical possibility for metastasized prostatic cancer is total prostatectomy. This operation is the choice of many urologists. It is done much like the prostatectomy for BPH, using either the retropubic or the perineal approach. These urologists feel that in removing the entire prostate, including the capsule itself, they surgically remove the entire cancer. However, these patients almost always lose their ability to have an erection. Today, however, there is hope for these men to continue an active sexual life. (Sexual functioning will be discussed fully in Chapter 9.)

If the cancer has spread beyond the capsule, sometimes total prostatectomy and bilateral orchidectomy are both recommended. If the adjacent lymph nodes have been invaded, these may also be removed.

RADIATION THERAPY

Radiation therapy is often used instead of, or in conjunction with, surgery and/or hormone therapy. If the cancer is limited to the prostate, radiation therapy may also be limited to the prostate. Treatments are given over a period of approximately six or seven weeks, usually in a clinic, hospital, or the specially equipped office of a radiotherapist. A machine is "aimed" at the patient, and the radiation is directed at the area selected by the radiotherapist in collaboration with the urologist. There is no pain or discomfort involved in the procedure; it's like having an ordinary x-ray picture taken. But the results can be dramatic, and radiotherapy can result in complete control of prostatic cancer, especially in the early stages. The treatment is prolonged over many weeks so that the doses can remain small in order to minimize reactions in the rectum and bladder, both very close to the prostate. Most reactions are unavoidable because radiation must go through these organs to reach the prostate. But reactions usually subside completely without any lasting effects.

If the tumor is a little more advanced and has spread beyond the prostate, the radiation would be directed toward the whole pelvic area in order to include all the pelvic nodes.

When the cancer has spread to the bones, radiation may be directed toward the area affected. This procedure minimizes pain and also helps a patient to avoid fractures that may result from even such relatively mild injuries as slipping on a wet pavement. Metastases from the prostate can cause weakening of the weight-bearing bones. Radiation can strengthen the bones, helping prevent such fractures.

Radiotherapists have contributed many new techniques to the treatment of prostatic cancer. Effective results are often obtained by concentrating the radiation within the prostate itself, thus sparing the surrounding tissues. In this method, a radiotherapist implants radioactive substances in the prostate to emit radiation locally.

At Mt. Sinai Medical Center in New York, Drs. Norman Simon and Sidney Silverstone implant very thin wirelike sources of radioactive cesium 137 in the prostate of certain patients. "Dummies" are implanted in the operating room, and later when the patient returns to his room, the inactive wires are replaced with active wires that have been stored in lead cylinder. The "dummies" are used, rather than "live," active wires so that no one in the operating room or elsewhere is exposed to radiation. Using these "dummies" allows for sufficient time to make any necessary adjustments (based on x-rays) to achieve accuracy in position. When the patient is back in the room the physician replaces these "dummy" wires quickly and efficiently. Protective measures are taken in the patient's room to avoid exposure to hospital staff and visitors. In a week the "live" wires are completely removed. Since the wires extend outside of the body, removal is a simple procedure.

Radioactive gold and iodine (I-125) isotopes can also be implanted directly into the prostate. This is also done in the operating room, but these remain in the prostate indefinitely, and are not removed.

Just as with external radiation, this internal radiation

must be very carefully calculated to avoid serious side effects on the rectum and on the bladder. The proper distribution of radioactive sources is of major importance, as is the calculation of the correct dosage. Other major medical centers now perform these procedures.

Given a choice, many patients prefer radiation—either external or internal—to surgery because there are fewer adverse effects on sexual activity. However, the risk that potency will be lowered does exist with radiation. So I advise a patient to base his decision on which method or methods will most likely affect the cancer and provide for a longer life. A urologist is best equipped to help a patient make that decision. I always try to remember that I am not just treating cancer of the prostate, but a *patient* with cancer of the prostate, and that the treatment depends on many variables.

A patient may have urinary blockage from the cancer, or benign prostatic hypertrophy (a distinct possibility because of his age) coexisting with the cancer. To afford him comfort and to prevent complications such as kidney failure, I will perform a TUR, as described earlier. However, I often wait a while until after cancer treatment has begun, because this treatment may sometimes also correct the BPH. If it doesn't, then I can do a TUR.

OTHER TREATMENTS

Aside from surgery, hormones, and radiation therapy, what else is available to the patient with cancer of the prostate? In some centers throughout the country, cryosurgery is being practiced. This technique involves the insertion of a probe of a very low temperature, which theoretically freezes and destroys the cancer. The studies of cryosurgery in treating cancer of the prostate are not sufficiently convincing to allow me to recommend this technique at this time, even for very small tumors. However, it may become the preferred treatment in the future.

Two other kinds of surgery are sometimes performed on patients with prostatic cancer. Hypophysectomy—removal of the pituitary gland—and adrenalectomy—removal of the adrenal glands—reduce the production of male hormones. At one time, removal of the pituitary gland required surgery through the skull, but today it is done through the upper gum and the nasal passage to the pituitary, which is located below the brain.

Dr. Ezra M. Greenspan, Clinical Professor of Medicine (Oncology) at the Mount Sinai School of Medicine, is optimistic over the improved potential of combination chemotherapy for cancer of the prostate. He says that chemotherapy (a combination of drugs given simultaneously or in sequence) has demonstrated dramatic results in other forms of cancer. However, chemotherapy with simultaneous estrogen therapy, when the estrogen (alone) fails to control the disease, has a definite place in the treatment of cancer of the prostate. Certain combinations of the new and older drugs are in the explorative stage, but encouraging results of increased survival are already emerging. The anticancer chemicals interfere with cancer cell growth and can also relieve symptoms. According to Dr. Greenspan, the use of these drugs requires a great deal of sophistication and involves some risk, so chemotherapy should be given under close supervision of a physician specifically trained in oncology.

Every few years, unproven cancer treatments are introduced and become available to the public. An example is the drug Laetrile. I am greatly opposed to the use of drugs that are unproven, or drugs administered without the careful supervision of doctors using established medical guidelines. Usually, detailed case histories are not published, nor do we see the initial results of treatment, as we do in established studies. Although many of these drugs do no harm by themselves, some *are* harmful, and believers often rely on them so heavily that they forego proven treatment. Too many people waste precious time and savings on such drugs when more reliable treatments are available. At this time, no diet has been proven to cure prostatic or any other kind of cancer.

The argument sometimes put forth that the medical profession and government agencies are not really interested in finding a cure for cancer is foolish. No doctor or government official is immune to cancer him- or herself, and most of my colleagues have, at some time, had cancer strike someone close to them. Doctors, like everyone else, hope to see cancer eradicated someday and are constantly reminding patients to seek diagnosis and treatment early.

For cancer of the prostate, early diagnosis and treatment is of great importance. The outlook for control of the disease is improving; of the approximately seventy thousand American men who will develop it during the next year, many will live to a ripe old age.

ZINC AND NUTRITION: EFFECTS ON THE PROSTATE

Patients often ask me if I think it would be helpful for them to take zinc pills, either to prevent prostate problems or to aid in the treatment of them. There is much controversy about the use of zinc as prevention or therapy for prostatic disease, so it is important to examine both sides of the question.

Zinc is a trace material found in all human beings. It is needed by the human organism in very small, almost microscopic amounts. However, deficiency of zinc can lead to major medical problems. Absence in childhood and adolescence can cause actual retardation of physical growth, delayed sexual development, impaired growth of hair, and roughness of skin. Any diet that supplies less than 10 milligrams a day is likely to cause some serious disturbances in the functioning of the body's organs and glands.

It has been noted for many years that zinc is found in high concentration in sperm, seminal fluid, and the prostate gland itself. The high zinc content of prostatic tissue has been noted by many researchers, and it has also been clearly demonstrated that the prostate contains more zinc than any other organ in the body. However, the reason for this high level of zinc in the prostate and its secretions is not known.

Studies on zinc and the prostate have been conducted

at many research centers, but no conclusive, universally acknowledged evidence has yet shown that if a man takes zinc pills, it will prevent or clear up his prostatic disease.

ZINC-PROSTATE STUDIES

At St. Louis's famous Washington University School of Medicine, Dr. William Fair, chairman of the Division of Urology, has long been interested in the relationship between zinc and the prostate. He states that zinc is important in the prevention of prostatic disease and may be important therapeutically as well. The only problem, he told me with disappointment, is that when zinc is administered orally, the prostate fails to pick it up. The zinc clearly gets into the bloodstream, but neither the prostatic tissue nor the prostatic fluid reap the benefits of the zinc tablets. Since the prostate doesn't get the zinc, it is unlikely that there will be any improvement or prevention of prostatic disease, even if a man persists in taking zinc tablets. However, Dr. Fair does state that he sees many patients who have taken zinc in foods or in capsule form report improvement in symptoms of either prostatitis or prostatism. But, he continues, these patients are also receiving some other kind of treatment, such as prostatic massage, so it is difficult to determine which treatment is helping. He agrees with many physicians who state that "whatever a doctor does within good reason and medical responsibility, some patients will get better, some will get worse, and some will remain the same." He also notes that there is a placebo effect at work. That is, if someone feels that something will make him feel better, it may indeed do that.

Dr. Fair is very optimistic about the future of zinc in treating prostatic disease. He states that zinc needs a carrier—that is, another substance that will guide the zinc to the prostate, where it can then work to prevent and alleviate symptoms. He informed my coauthor and me that he and his team of researchers are now working to identify a carrier molecule that can transport zinc to the prostate. It is possible, Dr. Fair says, that this carrier is something quite ordinary and that it is present in the diet of those men who have a favorable response to zinc.

Why are Dr. Fair and his researchers so interested in this rather complex relationship between zinc and the prostate? It is because they, like other researchers, have long noted that patients with chronic prostatitis have either a diminished amount or total absence of zinc in their prostatic secretion, as compared to men without prostatic problems. They feel that this suggests that the presence of zinc in the prostate may serve as a defense against prostatic and urinary infections. They have definitely found that, in vitro (in a test tube), the amount of zinc normally found in the prostatic fluid is effective against a variety of bacteria. At this time, Dr. Fair feels that there is some evidence that the drop in zinc concentration in prostatic fluid precedes any bacterial invasion of the prostate, rather than bacteria causing a drop in the zinc concentration. He and his team continue to pursue their studies on the relation between zinc and the prostate, in the hope that they will be able to use this information to benefit men everywhere.

Dr. Irving M. Bush, chairman of the Division of Urology at the Chicago Medical School, and his staff of researchers have also been studying zinc and its relation to the prostate. They have found that many men with prostatitis and benign prostatic hypertrophy were helped by the administration of oral zinc. Not only were symptoms reduced, but there was a shrinkage of the prostate in many of those patients with BPH.

Zinc also seems to be helpful in patients with congestive prostatitis, according to Dr. Bush. He feels that these patients' bodies don't have enough available zinc and, because the prostate is the place where most of the body's zinc is stored, conditions such as congestive prostatitis occur. There are, of course, individual differences in zinc needs. Diabetics, who need zinc for utilization of insulin, and heavy drinkers, who require zinc for breaking down alcohol in the liver—as well as individuals with other conditions not completely understood at this time—all have increased needs for zinc. Some doctors also believe that individuals undergoing unusual stress require additional zinc.

In these instances, the pituitary gland will send a message to the prostate saying "filter more zinc" and, in the prostate's effort to do this, congestion or enlargement of the glands may take place. The situation is also a bit like "borrowing from Peter to pay Paul." The zinc that is needed by other parts of the body is taken from the prostate, and then the prostate becomes zinc-starved. In an effort to manufacture more zinc, the prostate gets into trouble.

Dr. Bush explains that this pattern can be compared to thyroid conditions. The thyroid gland stores iodine, and if there is a shortage of iodine in the thyroid, the thyroid will enlarge. If iodine is administered to the patient early enough, the thyroid will shrink back to normal. If medical help is postponed, and the thyroid becomes greatly enlarged, the iodine may no longer be able to shrink the thyroid, but it will keep the gland from continuing to enlarge.

Dr. Bush finds that zinc therapy can also be helpful for BPH, if treatment is begun when the prostate is first beginning to enlarge. The zinc in the body, he explains, keeps the prostate glandular tissue from enlarging in order to produce zinc. Although zinc will not shrink the enlarged fibrous and muscular tissue, it *can* shrink the glandular tissue and afford the patient much relief. Since so many patients with BPH also have some form of prostatitis, the zinc will help this condition. Dr. Bush says patients report not only that they have a better sense of well-being from the combined zinc and vitamin therapy, but also that, because the glandular tissue shrinks, they urinate more comfortably and make far fewer "bathroom trips" at night. Dr. Bush says that he also continues the prostatic massage but finds that it becomes less necessary for many of these patients. Most important, he is avoiding surgery on an increasing number of these patients.

OBSERVING ZINC THERAPY

Dr. Bush told me that he reminds all of his patients that, although they are feeling much better and are showing fewer symptoms, it is essential that they be watched carefully. He continues to do diagnostic tests to test kidney function and, in addition, his patients have their semen and blood measured for zinc content. He also does regular semen cultures to check on bacteria.

In earlier studies, he only used zinc therapy on a patient for a few months, but he and his researchers have now moved beyond that initial work and are keeping patients on zinc therapy for longer periods of time. Some have already been on it for ten years. Dr. Bush says the zinc he prescribes has other vitamins and minerals included; he feels that this combination gives far better results than when zinc is used alone. He stresses that, while zinc may be ordinarily used in moderation by a patient along with regular daily vitamins, no man should try to prescribe zinc for himself to treat prostate problems. This must always be done under a doctor's supervision and, of course, every man over forty should have regular rectal examinations. If he is suffering from any prostatic symptoms, he should be given a thorough urological examination regularly, whether or not he is using zinc.

Many of my colleagues state that they have had patients ask them about zinc and, with their consent, the patients have begun a regimen of zinc tablets and a diet that includes zinc-rich foods. These patients often report a decrease in symptoms and, equally as important, a general sense of well-being. I have engaged in a study as well, and although it is less rigorous than Dr. Bush's, my results coincide with his.

ZINC-RICH FOODS

My patients are told to take zinc tablets, to eat zinc-rich foods, and to continue to see me regularly. I give prostatic massage and carefully watch the patients to be sure they are not having difficulties. It is my distinct impression that these patients are doing far better than the ones I used to treat with prostatic massage alone.

Foods that are rich in zinc include oysters, nuts, pumpkin seeds, sunflower seeds, wheat bran, wheat germ, brewer's yeast, milk, eggs, onions, molasses, chicken, peas, beans, lentil, beef liver, and gelatin. One of the problems in trying to rely upon diet to obtain zinc is that it is almost nonexistent in refined processed foods. Because of careless cooking and soil exhaustion, there are fewer high-zinc sources left to us than the above list would indicate. If the soil in which food grows is deficient in zinc—as much of it is—so will be the food. If the animals from which we obtain the food are also deficient in zinc, so will their products be deficient. To obtain natural zinc, it would be best to use garden-fresh (not just market-fresh) vegetables and to cook them slowly and at a low temperature. Although oysters are generally rich in zinc, the waters in which they live are often contaminated and the natural zinc has been diminished, if not altogether destroyed. In order for people to obtain the recommended daily allowance of 15 milligrams of zinc, it may be necessary to take zinc supplements. So if one is planning to use zinc as a protection against prostatic disease, or as an aid to therapy, it is probably necessary to take zinc supplements, rather than to rely on diet. However, as with any vitamin, mineral, or medication, one must remember the old adage about "too much of a good thing" and not take too much zinc. How much is too much? The amount varies with each individual and should be discussed with one's doctor. Most doctors seem to feel that an appropriate therapeutic dose is between 50 and 150 milligrams daily and that this dose is the maximum amount a patient can tolerate without any side effects. The side effects are seldom serious if checked in time but can be extremely uncomfortable. They may include diarrhea, nausea, and vomiting. One word of caution: there is some belief that large doses of zinc may diminish selenium (another metallic element) in the body, which some scientists believe may have a protective effect against cancer.

The foods that are rich in zinc have been used for thousands of years to treat various medical ills. As an aid to heal wounds, zinc has long been known to be effective, and present studies indicate that it has a definite place in the healing of chronic ulcers, burns, hepatitis, and wounds and may have a place in postsurgical healing. As yet its affect upon recovery from prostatic surgery has not been established, but studies are being conducted.

Pumpkin seeds, which are generally rich in zinc, have long been believed by many nutritionists and physicians to be effective in aiding prostatic health as well as sexual and neurological dysfunction. Almost fifty years ago, it was noted that BPH was almost nonexistent in Transylvania. Pumpkin seeds were an important part of the diet of the Translyvanians, and it is easy to draw the conclusion that there might be some relationship between their diet and the low incidence of BPH.

There are theorists who feel that zinc supplements may only be helpful if a deficiency already exists, but this has not been proven either. It is possible, of course, that some people's metabolism of zinc may be such that they require more than the usual amount to maintain prostatic health. In other words, an adequate amount of zinc for one man may be too little for another man, even if he doesn't have any special condition that would seem to require more zinc.

VITAMINS IN FOOD AND SUPPLEMENTS

Vitamin C is also thought by many nutritionists and physicians to be important in maintaining good prostatic health, and they recommend not only plenty of fresh vegetables and fruit in the diet, but supplementary Vitamin C as well. Vitamins A and D and Vitamin E are also considered important for prostatic health, and some experts believe that unsaturated fatty acids and pollen tablets may be helpful. Vitamins A, C, D, and E can of course be purchased as supplements in drug stores and health food stores, but many foods are also good sources for these vitamins. Foods rich in Vitamin A are calf and beef liver, chicken liver, spinach, turnip greens, cabbage, string beans, broccoli, carrots, yellow squash, apricots, sweet potatoes, and yams. Presence of Vitamin E is necessary to prevent destruction of Vitamin A, so the diet must include plenty of Vitamin E. The approximate daily requirement of Vitamin A for most adults is about 5,000 International Units, (I.U.) and anywhere from 10,000 to 20,000 I.U. can usually be consumed without any problems. Too much can cause a toxic effect, so more than the normal supplement of Vitamin A, as with all vitamins, should not be taken without close medical supervision.

Vitamin D is found in Vitamin D-enriched milk, fish liver oils, salmon, tuna, sardines, egg yolks, and margarine. Four hundred I.U. is the approximate daily requirement, and self-therapy should not include more than about 1,000 daily I.U. because serious toxic effect can result.

Vitamin E is found in wheat germ, whole grain bread and rice, safflower oil, vegetable oils, peanuts, and green leafy vegetables such as cabbage, spinach, asparagus, and broccoli. The approximate daily requirement for adults is 30 I.U. a day, and supplements should range from 30 to 100 I.U. Some nutritionists recommend up to 600 units a day, but since persons with high blood pressure, diabetes, or rheumatic heart should take only the minimum supplements, it would be wise to discuss this with a physician before embarking on a regimen of Vitamin E beyond the range of 30 to 60 I.U. per day.

Orange juice is best known as a supplier of Vitamin C, but broccoli, green pepper, brussels sprouts, strawberries, and cabbage also provide it—and with fewer calories. All citrus fruits and tomatoes are good sources of Vitamin C. The approximate daily requirement is 40 to 60 milligrams, but therapeutic doses range from 200 to 500 milligrams, although some nutritionists recommend even more. Excesses should be avoided because of the risk of forming kidney stones. Magnesium supplements should be taken along with large doses of Vitamin C, to aid in the prevention of this problem.

Essential fatty acids are also considered by many to be of importance in prostatic health. While the body can manufacture many of the fatty acids from carbohydrate and proteins, polyunsaturated fatty acids must be provided by foods. Hence they are often called essential fatty acids. Polyunsaturated fatty acids are found in vegetable oils and fish oils, and do not raise the body's cholesterol level. Essential fatty acid capsules, up to 1,200 milligrams per day, are thought by some nutritionists to be of therapeutic value in reducing the size of prostate enlargement. Other good food sources of fatty acids are unrefined seeds and whole grains, cold-pressed vegetable oils such as soybean oil, safflower oil, sunflower oil, and corn oil.

Lecithin, a substance found in egg yolks, is also considered important to prostatic health. Daily supplements of one to two tablespoons in granular, powder, or liquid form may be helpful.

Some studies in Sweden and Japan indicate that a pollen preparation called cernitin is very useful in treating prostatitis. Although I have had no experience with it, it seems to bear consideration. Pollen tablets are available at drug and health food stores; a recommended therapeutic dose is three tablets daily.

What one doesn't eat may be even more important than what one does eat, where prostatic health is concerned. It was noted earlier that spicy foods, coffee, and alcohol can have a deleterious effect on the prostate and should be avoided by those who already have prostatic problems. Others who are interested in prevention should consume these products with moderation. Zinc supplement may be extremely helpful to a man who does drink more beer or alcohol than he should because, as mentioned above, zinc can be helpful in alcohol breakdown in the liver.

Generally speaking, the rules of good nutrition apply to everyone, man, woman, and child. To the man who is reaching the age where prostatic problems are most likely to plague him, good diet is essential. Following some of the suggestions in this chapter may be extremely helpful. Although much of the value of zinc, vitamins, and diet to prostatic health is still in the exploratory stage and the statistics are not conclusive, the evidence is convincing enough for me to sit up and listen carefully, and I think others should do the same. However—and this is important in all self-care—never rely *only* on diet, vitamins, or minerals for good health. See your doctor regularly, even if you are feeling well. Before beginning on any new diet or regimen of vitamins, discuss it with him. A particular diet or vitamin dose may be clearly unwise for someone who has any other medical problem. It is best that a doctor know what his patient is taking and that he keep a record of it in the patient's chart. Then, if there should be any new symptoms, he can rule out the possibility of an allergy or toxic reaction to a vitamin or a new food, even if the dose taken is within the usual therapeutic range.

9

SEXUAL ACTIVITY AFTER PROSTATE SURGERY

Many years ago, when I was a young urologist and prostatic surgery was much more complicated and risky, an elderly patient was referred to me as a candidate for the operation. His life was in danger because of urinary blockage, but the man refused to consent to surgery until he fully discussed with me the effects the operation might have on his sexual activity. I had already taken a full medical, social, and sexual history from him, and I knew that this man had not engaged in sexual activity for many years. I wondered aloud why he was so concerned. He pointed out of the window at the Statue of Liberty and said, "See her over there? I haven't visited her in more than twenty years, but I do like knowing she's there."

His point was well made, and I never forgot it. I realized then that every man likes to know "it"—the ability to function sexually, when and if he wants to—"is still there."

Just about any man who is contemplating prostatic surgery worries about how the operation will affect his sex life. This is true regardless of whether the man has been sexually active or not, and regardless of whether he has a regular partner or is simply on the lookout for "Ms. Right."

For that reason, I always fully inform my patients concerning the possible effects of an impending prostatectomy upon sexual ability. Sometimes the patient's wife is the one who asks first about how the prostatectomy will affect her husband's sexual performance. In essence, my answer on that point is always the same; for the most part, if the man was able to engage in sex prior to surgery, he will be able to do so after surgery. If he couldn't or didn't before, the situation is not likely to change after surgery—at least not without special counseling or treatment.

My own experience with patients has been borne out in several studies done throughout the country. The type of surgery—whether TUR, suprapubic, or retropubic—is not a factor that affects changes in sexual functioning. For about 80 percent of men, after surgery sexual functioning returns to the presurgical level, about 10 percent improve, and about 10 percent lose some ability. Generally, those men who lose ability are in the oldest age group (over seventy), and most were only occasionally active prior to surgery.

When a change in sexual activity does accompany prostate problems or surgery for BPH, it is usually unrelated either to the condition or to the surgery itself. It is related instead to the age of the man, the way he views himself, and his life in general.

SEXUALITY IN LATER YEARS

The same incident can be perceived differently by different people, sometimes because of their individual personalities, but also because of their age difference. Trimming a Christmas tree or preparing the house for Passover gives people of all ages pleasure. The youngest usually focus on the doing and accomplishing. Middle-aged people tune in more to the sense of the holidays as well as the activity. The oldest take their time about it. They'll use an extra hour or so in trimming a tree, an extra day or so in preparing a house properly for Passover. But it's no more tiring, no less satisfying and, in many ways, much more pleasurable for them. All the meanings of the holiday—the remembrances of holidays past, the very appreciation of life lived to its fullest with people who mean a great deal, and the knowledge that life is fragile—contribute to a general sense of diffuse joy and pleasure that is often incomprehensible to the youngest participants.

This pleasure can be felt in many of the activities and experiences of the later years—sex for one. But too often people in their sixties and seventies decide that it's time to stop. If their sexual relationships were never good, they use advancing age as an excuse to stop. And maybe for them it is an answer. A sad answer, but maybe the right one if neither partner feels deprived. But for those who once took pleasure in loving and sex, age (in the absence of illness) is no reason to stop. Nor is prostatic surgery a reason to stop.

Older people have the capacity to function sexually and to enjoy it, but they need to know what physiological changes to expect with aging. Then they learn not only to compensate for these changes, but also to put them to advantage. A general slow-down in arousal and response are two of the most noticeable changes. These can affect and be affected by numerous other changes, too.

It takes men longer to become aroused and to achieve an erection than it did when they were young. Women may take longer to become comfortably lubricated. All too often, a couple misunderstand these signs. The husband thinks his ability to make love is almost gone, and his wife thinks she must have lost her allure. They wonder why it's taking him so long to get ready? When he does perform, why doesn't he ejaculate every time as before? And when he does ejaculate late, why does he lose his erection so rapidly? It's all normal; they just don't know it. He figures maybe something is wrong, but not with his wife; she still looks great.

So he has the family doctor check him out. No pain, no urinary problems. No need to see a urologist. The family doctor, who may be a nice young fellow, says to his patient, "Well, Jim, you are sixty-five. That happens." And Jim, who came in search of some sensible advice and reassurance that he's sexually okay, leaves with the feeling that he's on the verge of impotence.

Men who have had this type of experience often come to my office for some other reason. They might have BPH, totally unrelated to their recent sexual problems. We use my office consultation room to discuss their concerns.

I have discovered that most men are not aware that advancing age causes a definite slow-down in both the time it takes for sexual arousal and the time needed for ejaculation. The period of time it takes for them to achieve another erection (called the refractory period) is also longer than it once was. It's likely that an older man's erection will be less firm and will collapse almost immediately after ejaculation. There may be less force to his ejaculation. If a man is not prepared for these natural changes, of course he and his wife may become anxious.

For a man, *fear* of poor performance can *cause* poor performance, and is, in fact, the most frequent cause of impotence.

Those men who understand that these psychological changes are normal, and need not affect the quality or even quantity of sexual encounters, can relax and continue to enjoy their sexuality as it is.

Another change that accompanies the aging process is

the diminished urgency to ejaculate at the climax of every sexual experience. Still, the experience is satisfying and fulfilling. It is important that both partners realize this. Many men are also aware that it is possible to have an orgasm without ejaculation. That is, they might have the contractions of orgasm, and the satisfying pleasure that it brings, without having any emission of semen.

RETROGRADE EJACULATION

This brings us to an important phenomenon in physiological sexual activity following prostate surgery: retrograde ejaculation. Essentially, retrograde ejaculation occurs when the semen goes back into the bladder, rather than through the urethra and out of the penis. Sometimes a man is not even aware that this is happening until his partner calls his attention to it. She may think that he no longer "enjoys" sex, since he doesn't ejaculate. He may wonder if she's right, despite the pleasure he has experienced.

Prior to a TUR, a suprapubic, or a retropubic prostatectomy, I always explain to patients that retrograde ejaculation will probably result, for the following reason.

Ordinarily the bladder neck closes and the sphincter in the urogenital diaphragm opens at the time of orgasm, so that the sperm is driven down and out of the urethra and penis by the contracting muscles of the urethra. But after surgery, when the channel is sufficiently widened to allow the urine to flow, the bladder neck may be permanently open, causing the contractions of the muscles of the urethra to drive the semen upward through the open internal sphincter into the bladder. The fluid is then expelled when a man urinates after ejaculation. (After surgery, the available quantity of ejaculatory fluid will be diminished anyway because the source, the prostate gland, has been partially or completely removed.)

It is important to remember that retrograde ejaculation does not affect the sensation of orgasm, nor should it diminish the pleasure. However—and this is also important—it usually means that the man is infertile, or sterile. Men tend to confuse fertility with potency. Fertility and potency are independent of each other. A man capable of producing a large number of sperm is fertile, but he might, for physiological or psychological reasons, be unable to achieve an erection, in which case he is, by definition, impotent. Conversely, a man capable of achieving erection but unable to produce sperm, is sterile.

Because a man will probably have retrograde ejaculation after surgery for BPH, the sperm containing semen will not be deposited in his partner's vagina. Therefore, he is unlikely to impregnate her. However, a man whose partner is still of childbearing age should not depend on the retrograde ejaculation as a foolproof method of contraception. I always suggest that a man's ejaculate be examined in my office to see if he is still fertile; he must not presume that his prostate surgery will serve as a contraceptive.

To prevent epididymitis (inflammation of the epididymis), some urologists automatically perform a vasectomy (surgical cutting of the two vasa deferentia in the scrotum) when they remove a prostate. These patients will be sterile.

CAUSES OF IMPOTENCE

My reassurances to patients about resuming regular sexual activity after most prostate surgery (as discussed in

Chapter 6) will stand, and there should be few problems. But some people have problems anyway. Often they predate surgery. A careful history can sometimes reveal the reason. To determine whether a man's impotence or sexual dysfunction is caused by physiological or psychological reason I usually ask one simple question. Does he ever have an erection—in the morning, or during the night, or with masturbation? If the answer is yes, there is probably no physiological reason for the problem. However, there are many psychological explanations for why a man who was once sexually active becomes unable to achieve an erection sufficient for penetration.

Fear of poor performance is, as I said before, the most common reason. A man who is worried about how well he will do, and what his partner will think, is already in trouble. If he is worried about his partner's receptivity, he may also have problems. Masters and Johnson say that having an "interested and interesting partner" is vital to good sex. They also stress the importance of sexual regularity for aging men as a means of avoiding impotence. "Use it or lose it," they say. However, I have had patients who were sexually inactive for some time because of illness or lack of a partner, but who were able to resume activity when they recovered or found an "interested and interesting partner."

However, I never recommend abstinence as a way of preserving sexual ability. Contrary to some popular myths, there is no fixed quantity of sexual energy that can be used up, and the more consistently a man stays sexually active, the more likely he is to preserve his ability. The patient whom I described earlier as having been glad to see the Statue of Liberty out there, even though he didn't visit it, might still find she hasn't changed if he made a trip there, but if he waited too many years to check out his sexual ability, he would probably be in for a disappointment.

112

Some causes of impotence are physical, and some of them are reversible. Metabolic problems such as diabetes, or even a prediabetic state, are among the most common of these causes in older people. Impotence due to diabetes is not fully understood, but it is probably related in some way to damage to the neural pathways that send messages from spinal cord centers for erection. Such impotence is often unrelated to whether or not the diabetes is under control. A variety of medications can either reduce desire or cause impotence in this age group. Many drugs used for hypertension (high blood pressure) can cause difficulty with erections, but their effects tend to vary according to each individual. If a patient is affected adversely, the doctor can frequently give him another drug that will control the hypertension just as well, without having an unwelcome effect upon sexual ability. Digitalis, used for heart failure, can also cause sexual dysfunction.

Some of the drugs used as antidepressants tend to interfere with libido and sexual functioning even though they act as a stimulant for other activities. (But it should be noted that depressed individuals often have sexual problems anyway.)

Alcohol consumption commonly has an effect on sexual function. Chronic alcoholism will cause impotence in a man of any age, but for a man in his later years, even a few drinks too many may cause it.

COUNSELING CAN HELP

There are other causes of impotence in a man who was once sexually active—a problem called secondary impotence—and many men are amenable to treatment, whether the cause is physical or psychological. A thorough medical and urological checkup will often reveal physical reasons. If the cause is psychological, the patient and his partner may benefit from the reassurance a urologist can provide. Many people come to realize that the sexual slow-down can be like going to Europe on an ocean liner. Remember the slogan, "Getting there is half the fun?"

One of my patients realized this. His wife wrote me this letter—perhaps partly in fun:

> Dear Dr. Greenberger:
> Ever since you operated on my husband, it takes him almost a half hour of lovemaking to achieve an erection, and it's another ten minutes to orgasm. Before his surgery, it took him only five minutes of lovemaking to achieve an erection, and about one minute to have an orgasm. My sister wants to know if you can give her husband the same operation.

Of course, it wasn't the surgery that made the difference. It was simply the aging process that accompanied his BPH, and the benefits he had derived from his open discussion with me prior to and after surgery.

Other couples have learned that sexual activity does not necessarily mean sexual intercourse. It involves, rather, a whole sense of human sexuality. Holding, touching, mutual reaching out to each other physically is sex just as much as genital penetration is sex. And it can be just as satisfying. When people rid themselves of the idea that sexual activity which doesn't end with intercourse and orgasm is abnormal, they can fully understand their potential as sexual human beings.

When a patient does not respond to the information or the reassurances I offer, I often refer him to someone like my coauthor, who is a trained and experienced counselor. She describes one such case:

One couple I counseled about sexual difficulties stands out in my mind. I met him first. He was a lawyer, still in active practice—handsome, grey-haired, age sixty-eight. He had a mischievous grin, but his eyes were sad. As he told me about himself, I could see that he was intelligent and highly creative. His wife, an attractive woman, had been a teacher. Together they had brought up two daughters, one a journalist, the other a lawyer like her father.

For the last seven years this couple had had no sexual contact. None at all. He told it to me this way:

"About seven years ago, I had a prostate operation. Before that our sex life had been just so-so. Sex was just a once-in-a-while thing. After my operation, I felt better than ever. The doctor assured me surgery shouldn't affect my sexual ability. However, the first time we tried, I just couldn't get an erection. The second time was the same. And the third time. I haven't tried since."

"How do you feel about this?" I asked.

"It's not so much the sex act that I miss," he answered. "I miss the touching, the holding, the physical contact. I miss it very much."

In the course of our interviews, I obtained a full history of this couple, and I was able to put together the whole picture.

At one time, they had had a happy and satisfying sex life. But it was mostly focused on performance. He found his wife exciting and took great pride in the fact that he could always get ready quickly. She was flattered and happy that she could elicit this response in him, and much of the time she responded to their lovemaking with enthusiasm, if not always with orgasm. There were times when she didn't much feel like having sex, but she remembered her mother's wedding advice: "If *you* don't, there's always some other woman who will."

So their sex life, never really as full as it might have been, had deteriorated to the point of nonexistence. The husband admitted that it was not only that he missed their old relationship, but that he also wanted what they

115

had never really had. His wife, in separate interviews with me, said much the same thing.

Their lack of communication and the husband's fear of performance had driven them apart sexually, although they still had much in common and shared many good times together. As our sessions continued and the channels of communication opened up, both were able to speak freely about their current sex life and what they wanted it to be. The husband confessed that he was afraid if he aroused his wife and then couldn't perform, she would be frustrated and angry. When his wife heard this, she reminded him that penetration is possible even without a full erection, and she said that she could also reach orgasm if he caressed her sexually sensitive areas. Not only was this lady thoughtful and considerate, but apparently she had also been reading some sex-counseling literature. She opened the door for her husband to just enjoy the sensual experience of lovemaking. She relieved him of any demand to "perform" so that he did not have to worry about success or failure.

The above case is more common than many people realize. Although fear of failure will lead to sexual dysfunction in both men and women, it is particularly true for men. Women can perform sexually without arousal; men can't.

A CURE FOR IMPOTENCE

A man who has been adversely affected by surgery either for BPH or for cancer of the prostate, or who has experienced reduced libido or ability to achieve erection because he is taking estrogens for cancer of the prostate, can still participate in a sexual experience. He, like the aging man who has occasional or even chronic trouble achieving a full erection, knows that there must have been many occasions when his wife wasn't really "in the mood" but took pleasure in his pleasure. He can now do the same for her and find that his lovemaking, manual or oral as well as genital, can give her much pleasure and satisfaction. In turn, it can give him the same kind of pleasure and satisfaction he experienced in earlier years. For those men who feel there is no substitute or alternative to achieving an erection firm enough for vaginal penetration, there is an option. For the last ten years, it has been possible to successfully implant into the penis a solid or inflatable object that permits a satisfactory erection. There are three available kinds of penile prostheses (as these are called). Some urologists have a preference for one of these types, but others offer a choice to their patients.

The Small-Carrion Penile Prosthesis, developed by Dr. Michael P. Small and Dr. Herman M. Carrion of the University of Miami School of Medicine, consists of silicone tubes containing spongy material. It is surgically inserted into the penis and provides the man with a flexible semi-rigid penis. It enables him to have satisfactory intercourse, but since he now has a permanent erection, he may find it is embarrassing to wear tight clothes or a bathing suit. This prosthesis is the one my associates and I recommend, and we find that most of the post-total-prostatectomy patients who consider it don't wear tight jeans or bikini bathing suits anyway, so they are not troubled by the problem of embarrassment.

The Flexi-Rod Penile Implant, a more recent development, is similar to the Small-Carrion, but it is made with flexible rods, so it enables the penis to hang more naturally and is usually not noticeable when a man is dressed, even in slim-line clothes. This prosthesis permits satisfactory intercourse, but it is a little more difficult to achieve penetration than with the Small-Carrion.

The Inflatable Penile Prosthesis is being implanted by many urologists. It simulates a natural erection and, according to Dr. F. Brantley Scott of the Baylor College of Medicine in Houston, Texas, requires a relatively simple technique to implant. Hollow cylinders are implanted in the penis and are filled with water by means of a silicone rubber pump placed under the scrotum. Based on a simple procedure using a cylinder, pump, reservoir, and interconnecting tubes, it is all concealed under the skin and cannot be seen from the outside. Not all urologists have received special training in using this prosthesis, but there are many urologists across the country who do use it competently. At Beth Israel Hospital in New York, Dr. Arnold Melman, physician-in-charge for the Center for Male Sexual Dysfunction, told me that he leaves the choice of prosthesis to the patient, after fully describing and demonstrating them.

In my opinion, this surgery has a definite place in the collaborative disciplines of medicine, psychiatry, and social work. I believe that no man should consider it without full exploration of his feelings about sexual functioning, his reason for wanting the surgery, and his expectation of what this will mean in his life. If he has a wife or regular partner, the decision must be a joint one. Frequently, a man decides he wants a penile implant to please his partner, only to find out later that the partner would not have made this decision if consulted about it prior to surgery.

I believe—and most of the sexual counselors and urologists with whom I have discussed this issue agree— that there should be a joint discussion with both partners. Some urologists refer *all* patients contemplating this surgery to a competent sexual counselor, prior to and even after surgery.

But for many who are either having difficulty or are unable to obtain an erection sufficient for penetration, a prosthesis is not the answer. For them, loving and caring and sexuality are not necessarily dependent on sexual intercourse; for these men and their partners, a penile prosthesis implant is not an option they choose.

NEVER TOO LATE

When people view sexuality as a shared mutual experience, the giving to each other of emotional and physical satisfaction without any specific goal in mind, they can find greater pleasure in life. Unfortunately, their grown children, the media, and some physicians tend to look at older folks with amusement or even disdain when they see them showing signs of anything more than mild affection. But most doctors and counselors who treat people of all ages know that sexuality and sexual desire can last a lifetime and are the norm rather than the exception.

It is not my intention to provide a "cookbook" approach to achieving sexual success after prostatectomy or at any particular age or stage of life. I only want to convey my profound conviction that it's never too late to enjoy sexual activity. Of course, physiological changes occur with aging, as well as with surgery or treatment, but they need not diminish the pleasure we can take in our sexuality.

119

GLOSSARY

abscess a collection of pus, often resulting in swelling, fever, and pain.

ampulla a small dilation in a canal or duct.

androgens hormones that encourage the development and maintenance of male sex characteristics. Testosterone is an androgen. Absence of androgens will usually cause the prostate to shrink.

anesthetic a substance that causes loss of sensation in all or part of the body. General anesthetic causes lack of consciousness and sensation. Local anesthetic causes only lack of sensation.

antihistamine any of the drugs used to relieve the symptoms of allergies and colds. Antihistamines work by neutralizing the effects of histamine, an active substance in allergic reactions.

anus the opening found at the end of the digestive tract, through which waste products are excreted.

121

aspiration

the removal by suction of air, fluid, or tissue from an area in the body.

atrophy

the emaciation, shrinking, or wasting of tissues, organs, or the entire body for any of a number of possible causes. For example, a man's testes will atrophy (although the scrotum will remain intact) if he is deprived of male hormones or given female hormones.

bacteria

a broad class of one-celled microorganisms, some of which must live and feed off other living things. Many, but not all, bacteria are capable of causing disease.

benign

a term used to characterize a mild illness or a nonmalignant growth. Thus, a benign (or nonmalignant) tumor is one that does not invade and destroy neighboring normal tissue.

benign prostatic hypertrophy (BPH)

the enlargement or growth of the glandular tissue within the prostatic capsule. Does not spread or attack other tissue or cells, but can push prostate outward, thus narrowing the bladder outlet.

bilateral

possessing or related to two sides.

biopsy

a procedure whereby tissue is removed from living patients so that it can be further studied and aid the physician in making a medical diagnosis.

122

bladder

in medical usage, the urinary bladder, an elastic sac that serves to store urine before it is excreted from the body.

blood acid phosphatase level

the measure of relative amount of phosphatase in blood. Phosphatase is an enzyme found in almost all tissues, body fluids, and cells. An increase of acid phosphatase in the blood may indicate cancer of the prostate, as well as other diseases.

blood alkaline level

the measure of relative amount of substances capable of neutralizing acids. They play an important role in maintaining normal functioning of the body.

bone marrow

the soft, spongelike material found inside the cavities of bones. It is here that red blood cells, white blood cells, and platelets are made.

bone scan

a picture of the bones obtained by first injecting the patient with a radioactive chemical that travels to the areas around the bone, thus highlighting any bone injury, repair, or bone destruction. The bone scan is an extremely sensitive test, particularly useful in the diagnosis of prostate cancer that may have metastasized to the bones.

bone survey

a complete series of x-rays of the skeletal system. This survey is used as a diagnostic aid in detecting cancer.

cancer   the uncontrolled growth of abnormal cells. Also called malignant neoplasm or malignancy.

candida albicans   a type of yeastlike fungus that usually causes infection of the throat, vagina, and gastrointestinal tract. If left unchecked, it can sometimes lead to more serious disease.

cardiovascular   relating to circulation, to the heart and blood vessels.

castration   in men, the removal of testicles by surgery, or suppression of male hormones by administration of female hormones.

catheter   a hollow, flexible tube designed to be passed through the urethra into the bladder in order to drain urine.

cauterization   the burning or scarring of skin or tissue by the use of heat, chemicals, or instruments. Usually done to destroy abnormal tissue.

chemotherapist   a physician especially trained in the use of chemotherapy.

chronic   continuous or of long duration. Certain diseases are chronic in that they slowly progress and/or continue for long periods of time.

coitus   sexual intercourse.

coitus interruptus	conscious withdrawal of the penis during intercourse prior to ejaculation and/or orgasm.
coitus prolongus	conscious postponement of ejaculation and/or orgasm during intercourse.
complete blood count	the number of blood cells in a given sample of blood. Counting the number of different blood cell types aids in the diagnosis of disease.
congestion	swelling due to the presence of increased blood in blood vessels or tissues.
contraceptive	any drug, device, or method designed to prevent pregnancy.
Cowper's glands (or bulbourethral glands)	two glands located on either side of the male urethra. They produce a secretion that becomes part of the seminal fluid.
cryosurgery	surgery with the use of extremely low temperature.
crystallization	the process of a gas or liquid becoming a solid, thus forming a crystal.
cunnilingus	sexual stimulation of the female genitals by mouth or tongue.
cystoscope	a lighted instrument which is passed through the urethra and into the bladder for examination of the bladder interior.

diabetes — generally, a chronic disease caused by deficiency of insulin, which results in an inability of the body to utilize starches and sugars. The disease is characterized by excess sugar in the blood and urine, water loss, weakness, and a decrease of alkaline substances in urine relative to the amount of acids. Some forms of diabetes are mild and respond well to diet and/or or oral medication; other forms are more severe and can cause complications if not controlled by insulin injections as well as diet.

diagnosis — the process of determining the nature of a disease. It is a necessary preliminary to treatment.

dilation (also dilitation) — the widening or stretching of a body passageway that is malfunctioning due to a narrowing, accomplished by the insertion of progressively thicker instruments. Dilation of the urethra is frequently necessary when strictures develop.

distention — the swelling, stretching, or expansion of a body part, often resulting from an accumulation of gas or fluid.

diverticulum (plural, diverticula) — a pouch or sac that opens from a hollow organ such as the urethra or bladder.

dysfunction   difficult or abnormal functioning of an organ or body part.

ejaculation   the discharge or expulsion of semen from the penis, usually—but not necessarily—accompanied by orgasm. The ejaculate fluid, or semen, consists of sperm and other secretions.

ejaculatory ducts   tubes connected to seminal vesicles. They run through the prostate gland and are involved in the ejaculatory process.

electrocardiogram (EKG or ECG)   a graphic record or tracing of the actions of various portions of the heart. The instrument used for the recording is an electrocardiograph, and the graphic record it produces is used in the diagnosis of heart disease.

enuresis   bedwetting or involuntary passage of urine, usually at night or during sleep.

enzyme   a protein substance that can induce changes in other substances without changing its own characteristics.

epididymis (plural, epididymides)   a long, convoluted structure along the border of each testicle. Sperm is stored in the ducts of the epididymides until it reaches full maturity.

epididymitis inflammation of the epididymis.

erection the enlargement and stiffening of the penis when it becomes filled with blood as a result of sexual stimulation.

estrogens a general name for female sex hormones. They are made in the ovaries and, although each hormone has a slightly different function, they are closely related and usually referred to collectively as "estrogen." Estrogen is responsible for the development of reproductive organs and secondary sex characteristics of the female. Synthetic estrogens are used in the treatment of prostatic cancer and in many treatments for conditions in women.

excretion the process whereby undigested food and waste products are eliminated from the body.

fascia a band or sheet of tissue that covers the muscles and various organs of the body, below the skin.

fellatio sexual stimulation of the penis by mouth or tongue.

fertile capable of conceiving and bearing children.

foreskin (or prepuce) the free fold of skin that covers, more or less completely, the head of the penis. The foreskin is partially or totally removed in circumcision.

genitals (or genitalia)	the male and female reproductive organs, both internal and external.
gland	a collection of cells forming an organ that produces or manufactures material which may be secreted into the bloodstream or excreted outside the body.
glans	(male) an acorn-shaped structure, the "glans penis" refers to the tip of the penis. (female) the "glans clitoridis" refers to the small mass of erectile tissue at the tip of the clitoris.
gynecologist	a physician who specializes in diseases, reproductive physiology, and endocrinology of females.
gynecomastia	excessive enlargement and development of breasts.
hematologist	a physician who specializes in problems of the blood and bone marrow.
hematuria	any condition in which the urine contains blood or red blood cells.
hemospermia	presence of blood in the seminal fluid.
history, medical	a record of past illness, operations, accidents, and other relevant experiences of the patient. A history may also include information about the patient's family and forebears.
impotence	inability in the male to achieve and maintain an erection sufficient for penetration.

incontinence   inability to prevent discharge of urine or feces.

infection   usually, the invasion and multiplication of certain diseases caused by microorganisms.

inflammation   a condition resulting from injury, infection, or irritation. The common signs of inflammation are redness, heat, swelling, and pain.

intravenous pyelogram (IVP)   a series of x-ray pictures taken after the intravenous injection of dye into the patient's bloodstream. These x-ray pictures outline the urinary bladder, ureters, and kidneys. The dye is excreted by the kidneys. Also referred to as *intravenous urography*.

kidneys   two bean-shaped organs located on each side of the spinal column. Blood passes through them, and the impurities that are removed there dissolve and form urine.

libido   conscious or unconscious sexual desire.

lithology   study or science of rocks or calcium stones.

lymph node   one of many round or oval bodies placed at strategic points in the body. They supply the blood with lymphocytes (a type of white blood cell) and in turn remove bacteria and foreign matter from the lymph. This filtering-out of infection serves to protect the body.

malignancy   see cancer.

masturbation   the stimulation or manipulation of one's own or another's genital organs for sexual gratification.

metabolism   all those physical and chemical processes involved in the maintenance of life and which result in tissue change. Basically, these processes are of two types: those that involve the breaking down of larger particles into smaller ones and thereby produce energy; and those that convert small particles into larger ones, and thereby use up energy.

metastasis   the shifting, spread, or colonization of an original cancerous tumor to another part of the body. It is usually transported through the bloodstream or lymph system.

metstatic lesion   a small patch of malignant tissue, or tumor, that has spread from the original site of cancer, however remote.

microscopic   too small to be visible to the naked eye, but large enough to be visible under a microscope.

neoplasm   a tumor, or abnormal new growth or swelling of tissue. It can be either benign or malignant.

nephritis   acute or chronic inflammation of the kidneys.

nocturia   the urge or need to urinate at night.

nocturnal emission
a discharge of seminal fluid during sleep. It may be the result of erotic dreams, or simply a natural way to rid the body of accumulated sperm and secretions. Often referred to as a "wet dream."

nodule
a small mass of tissue or a tumor, generally malignant.

oncologist
a physician specifically trained to treat neoplasms or tumors.

oncology
the study, science, or treatment of neoplasms and tumors.

oral genital sex
sexual stimulation of the genitals by the mouth or tongue (see fellatio and cunnilingus).

orchidectomy
the surgical removal of one or both testicles. When an orchidectomy is performed for cancer of the prostate, the scrotum is left intact.

orgasm
the climax of the sexual act, usually accompanied by muscular contractions, release of tension, and pleasurable sensation. In men orgasm is usually, but not always, accompanied by ejaculation. Orgasm may occur without erection.

pathology
the part of medicine that deals with all aspects of disease, particularly with the nature, causes, and development of the disease state and the changes that accompany it.

132

pelvic congestion (female) during sexual stimulation a woman's pelvic organs become flooded with arterial blood. During orgasm the involuntary muscular contractions block further arterial blood from entering the pelvic area and draining off any remaining blood. If a woman is consistently aroused sexually without reaching orgasm, the pelvic blood vessels do not empty and remain congested and engorged with stagnant blood. This results in uncomfortable chronic pelvic congestion.

pelvis the lower part of the body formed by the two hip bones and the lower portion of vertebral column, constituting the lowest part of the trunk.

penis the male organ which serves for urinary excretions and for sexual intercourse.

perineal prostatectomy the removal of all or part of the prostate gland through an incision in the perineum, the area between the anal opening and the scrotum.

pituitary gland an endocrine gland located at the base of the brain. It produces hormones that regulate secretions of other endocrine glands.

potency the ability of a man to achieve and maintain an erection sufficient for penetration.

prepuce   see foreskin.

prognosis   the doctor's forecast of the probable outcome of a disease.

prostate   the male gland which surrounds the urethra. It secretes fluid which forms part of the semen that is expelled during ejaculation.

prostatism   acute, chronic, or temporary inflammation of the prostate gland, usually caused by infection, congestion, or irritation.

pubis   the area just above external genitals.

radiation   the process of emitting radiant energy in the form of x-rays, electromagnetic, light, short radio, ultraviolet, or any other rays from one source or center. In medicine, these rays are used for purposes of treatment or diagnosis.

radiotherapist   a physician who is specially trained in radiotherapy.

radiotherapy   the use of electromagnetic rays, or radiation, in the treatment of disease.

rectum   the end portion of the large intestine extending from the sigmoid colon to the anal canal.

red blood cells minute, disk-shaped blood cells that float in the blood and contain hemoglobin. They are responsible for the color of the blood, the transport of oxygen to the tissues and of carbon dioxide away from the tissues.

refractory period — the amount of time a man requires after ejaculation and/or orgasm before he is able to achieve a second erection.

resectoscope — an instrument inserted through the urethra during surgery. It is used for the removal of all or part of the prostate gland during a transurethral resection, as well as in other surgical procedures in both men and women.

retrograde ejaculation — the flow of semen backwards into the bladder instead of forward through the penis. A frequent result of prostate surgery.

retrograde pyelogram — an x-ray picture of the ureters and kidneys that is taken after dye is introduced into the ureters by way of catheters.

retropubic prostatectomy — surgical removal of all or part of the prostate gland through an incision in the lower abdomen, below the navel and slightly above the penis. The bladder is not opened in this procedure.

scrotum — the external sac of skin that contains the testicles.

secretion
a substance that is produced by a cell, or group of cells, of an organism and stored or utilized by that organism.

seminal fluid (or semen)
a thick, yellowish-white fluid that contains spermatozoa. It is a mixture of secretions from the testicles, the seminal vesicles, the prostate gland, and the Cowper's glands.

seminal vesicles
two folded glandular structures that lie against the lower rear bladder wall. The secretions of the seminal vesicles form part of the semen.

serum
the fluid portion of the blood that is obtained after the blood cells and fibrin clot have been removed.

sexual dysfunction
inability to achieve sexual relations that will result in satisfaction and/or orgasm.

sperm (or spermatozoa)
the male sex cell, or gamete (composed of a head and a tail), that fertilizes the ovum (female sex cell). Within the spermatozoa is the genetic information that will be transmitted to offspring. Sperm forms part of the semen ejaculated from the penis.

sphincter
a ringlike muscle whose relaxation or contraction regulates the amount of substance that can pass through a tube or out of an organ.

sterile	unable to produce offspring.
sterilization	the process by which a person is made incapable of producing offspring.
stilbestrol	a synthetic female hormone, frequently given to patients with cancer of the prostate.
stricture	a narrowing of a structure or passageway.
suprapubic prostatectomy	the removal of all or part of the prostate gland through an incision made in the skin below the navel and slightly above the pubis in the lower abdomen. The bladder is opened in this procedure.
suture	surgical stitches bringing together two surfaces.
testicles (or testes; singular, testis)	the two male reproductive glands that produce sperm and androgens. They are enclosed in the scrotum.
testosterone	a hormone that encourages the development and maintenance of male sex characteristics.
total prostatectomy	surgical removal of the entire prostate gland and capsule.
transurethral resection	surgical removal of all or part of the prostate gland by means of passing an instrument through the penis and urethra to cut away tissue in the prostate gland.

tumor	swelling or enlargement due to abnormal overgrowth of tissue. Neoplasm is a term used to refer to tumors that are composed of new and actively growing tissue. Their growth is faster than that of normal tissue and serves no useful purpose. Tumors can be either benign or malignant.
umbilicus (navel or belly button)	the point in the center of the abdomen marking the spot where the umbilical cord originally entered into the body when it was a fetus.
uremia	an excess of urea and other nitrogenous wastes in the blood.
ureter	the long, narrow tube through which the urine passes from the kidney to the bladder.
urethra	in men and women, the muscular tube or canal through which the urine passes from the bladder out of the body. In men, seminal fluid as well as urine passes through the urethra.
urine	fluid that is excreted by the kidneys, stored in the bladder, and expelled through the urethra. Urine consists of 96 percent water and 4 percent dissolved substances.
urology	the study, diagnosis, and treatment of diseases of the male genitourinary tract and female urinary tract.

vagina   the female genital canal.

varicocele   a varicose condition of the veins of the spermetic cord, causing a benign, boggy tumor of the scrotum.

vas deferens (plural, vasa deferentia)   one of the two tubes attached to the epididymis, extending to the prostatic urethra, and looping behind the bladder, where it becomes the ejaculatory duct.

vasectomy   the removal of a part of the vas deferens. Bilateral vasectomy results in sterility.

venereal disease   a type of disease relating to or resulting from sexual relations. (However, not all diseases related to sex are V.D.).

white blood cells   minute cell bodies in the blood (about one-third larger than the red cells) that act against infection.

work-up   a term that covers medical examination and tests, often done in a hospital, to arrive at a diagnosis and complete medical picture of the patient.

FOR FURTHER READING

American Society of Hospital Pharmacies. *Consumer Drug Digest*. New York: Facts on File, Inc., 1982.

Belsky, Marvin S., M.D., and Gross, Leonard. *How to Choose and Use Your Doctor*. New York: Arbor House, 1979.

Better Homes and Gardens After-Forty Health and Medical Guide. Better Homes and Gardens, 1980.

Better Homes And Gardens Books Editor, ed. *New Family Medical Guide,* revised ed. Better Homes and Gardens, 1982.

Brody, Jane. *Jane Brody's Nutrition Book*. New York: W. W. Norton & Co., 1981. Bantam paper, 1982.

Brody, Jane. *Jane Brody's The New York Times Guide to Personal Health*. New York: Times Books, 1982.

Brooks, Marvin B. *Lifelong Sexual Vigor: How to Avoid and Overcome Impotence*. New York: Doubleday, 1981.

Butler, Robert N., M.D., and Lewis, Myrna I., A.C.S.W. *Sex After Sixty: A Guide for Men and Women for Their Later Years*. New York: Harper and Row, 1976. (In paper, entitled *Love and Sex After Sixty: A Guide for Men and Woman for Their Later Years*. New York: Harper and Row, 1977.)

Carrera, Michael. *Sex: The Facts, the Acts and Your Feelings*. New York: Crown, 1981.

Comfort, Alex, M.D. *The Joy of Sex*. New York: Crown, 1972. Fireside/Simon and Schuster paperback, 1976.

Corsaro, Maria and Korzeniowsky, Carole. *STD: A Commonsense Guide to Sexually Transmitted Diseases*. New York: Holt Rinehart & Winston, 1982.

Farrell, Michael P., and Rosenberg, Stanley D. *Men at Midlife*. Boston: Auburn House, 1981.

Glabman, Sheldon, M.D., and Freese, Arthur S. *Your Kidneys, Their Care and Their Cure*. New York: Dutton, 1976.

Good Housekeeping Family Health and Medical Guide. New York: Hearst Books, 1980.

Harrington, Geri. *The Medicare Answer Book*. New York: Harper and Row, 1982. (Publisher will send free Medicare update which will list any major new developments that occur.)

Harrington, Geri, and Harrington, Ty. *Never Too Old*. New York: Times Books, 1981.

Herink, Richie, ed. *The Psychotherapy Handbook*. New York: New American Library, 1980.

Isenberg, Seymour, and Elting, L. M. *The Consumer's Guide to Successful Surgery*. New York: St. Martin's Press, 1976.

Johnson, G. Timothy, M.D., and Goldfinger, Stephen E., M.D. *The Harvard Medical School Health Letter Book*. Cambridge, MA: Harvard University Press, 1981. Warner paperback, 1982.

Jones, Judith K. ed. *Good Housekeeping Family Guide to Medications*. Hearst Books, 1980.

Landers, Ann. *The Ann Landers Encyclopedia A to Z*. New York: Doubleday, 1978. Ballantine paperback, 1979.

Lyons, Albert S., M.D., and Petrucelli, R. Joseph II, M.D. *Medicine: An Illustrated History*. New York: Harry N. Abrams, 1978.

Michaels, Joseph. *Prime of Your Life: A Practical Guide to Your Mature Years*. New York: Facts on File, Inc., 1981.

Morra, Marion, and Potts, Eve. *Choices: Realistic Alternatives in Cancer Treatment*. New York: Avon, 1980.

Nourse, Alan E., M.D. *Ladies Home Journal Family Medical Guide*. New York: Harper and Row, 1973.

Nirenberg, Judith, R.N., and Janovic, Florence. *The Hospital Experience: A Complete Guide to Understanding and Par-*

ticipating in Your Own Care. New York: Bobbs-Merrill, 1978.

Pinckney, Cathey, and Pinckney, Edward, M.D. *The Encyclopedia of Medical Tests.* New York: Facts on File, Inc., 1982.

Rosenfeld, Isador, M.D. *The Complete Medical Exam,* New York: Simon and Schuster, 1978.

Rothenberg, Robert E., M.D. *New Understanding Surgery: The Complete Surgical Guide.* New York: New American Library, 1976.

Rothenberg, Robert E., M.D. *The New American Medical Dictionary and Health Manual.* New York: Crown, 1975. Revised paper edition: New American Library.

Rothenberg, Robert E., M.D. *Health in the Later Years.* New York: New American Library, 1972.

Silber, Sherman J., M.D. *The Male from Infancy to Old Age.* New York: Scribner, 1981.

Starr, Bernard D., and Weiner, Marcella Bakur. *The Starr-Weiner Report on Sex and Sexuality in the Mature Years.* New York: Stein and Day, 1981.

Waller, Kal. *How to Recover Your Medical Expenses.* New York: Macmillan, 1981.

Wyndner, Ernest L., M.D., ed. *The American Health Foundation's The Book of Health.* New York: Franklin Watts, 1981.

INDEX

145